Encyclopedia of Natural Health Secrets and Cures

by Janice McCall Failes and Frank W. Cawood

Acknowledgments

To Betty Whitfield, Wanda Jennings and Gayle Cawood, for your thorough editing and insights.

To Andrew Aronfy, M.D., for your critical review and suggestions.

To Linda Sciullo, for your faithfulness, constant encouragement and endless patience.

To Debbie Williams, for your artwork and design.

To all the staff of FC&A, for your support and willingness to help.

To the people of Beth Horon and Mount Olivet United Methodist churches and the Rockbridge/Augusta Christian Writers' Group in Virginia, who have provided prayerful support throughout the research and writing of this book.

To our spouses, Gayle and Walter B., for your constant encouragement and abiding love.

Our thanks and praise is for our Lord and Savior, who created us, heals us and gives us eternal life.

Praise the Lord!
For it is good to sing praises to our God;
For it is pleasant and praise is becoming.
The Lord builds up Jerusalem;
He gathers the outcasts of Israel.
He heals the brokenhearted,
And binds up their wounds.

— Psalm 147: 1-3
New American Standard Translation

Is anyone amoung you sick? Let him call
for the elders of the church, and let them
pray over him, anointing him with oil in the
name of the Lord; and the prayer offered
in faith will restore the one who is sick,
and the Lord will raise him up, and if he
has committed sins, they will be forgiven
him.
Therefore, confess your sins to one
another, and pray for one another, so that
you may be healed. The effective prayer of
a righteous man can accomplish much.

— James 5: 14-16
New American Standard Translation

Table of Contents

Introduction 9

Allergy Relief 11
Alzheimer's Disease 17
Appendicitis 21
Arthritis 22
Asthma 29
Back Pain 31
Bedwetting 32
Bites By Insects 32
Blood Pressure — High 34
Bronchitis 38
Cancer 40
Child Care 60
Cholesterol Reduction 60
Cold Sensitivity 68
Colds 72
Constipation 77
Dandruff 79
Dental Problems 80
Depression 84
Diabetes 90
Diarrhea 90

Endometriosis 91
Epilepsy 93
Exercise 94
Eye Problems 95
Falls 98
Feminine Hygiene 100
Fertility (See Infertility) 102
Fibrocystic Breast Disease 102
Food Poisoning 103
Foot Problems 109
Gas 111
Gum Disease 112
Hair Care 114
Hair Loss In Women 114
Headaches 116
Hearing Problems 119
Heart Problems 120
Heat Stress 127
Hoarseness 131
Hyperactivity 132
Indigestion 133
Infertility 134
Kidney Problems 135
Lead Poisoning 136
Leg Pain 140
Memory Loss 141
Osteoporosis 142

Ovarian Cysts 143
Pain 144
Pregnancy 145
Premenstrual Syndrome (PMS) 150
Pressure Sores 154
Safe Sex 156
Skin Problems 156
Sleep Problems 166
Sneezing 173
Stress 174
Stroke 177
Sunburn 178
Sunstroke 179
Swimmer's Ear 180
Taste — Loss of 181
Teeth (See Dental Problems) 182
Toxic Shock Syndrome (TSS) 182
Ulcers 183
Vocal Problems (See Hoarseness) 184
Weight Loss Tips 184
Wrinkles (See Skin Problems) 192

Introduction

As the amount of medical knowledge in our world is increasing, we saw the need for a straightforward book, written in everyday English, to help us understand how medical research can change our lives. <u>Encyclopedia</u> <u>of</u> <u>Natural</u> <u>Health</u> <u>Secrets</u> <u>and Cures</u> is that book. It has been written to simply explain some of the fascinating tips that can easily be used for a naturally healthier life.

Many of the suggestions reported may be controversial or unproven by controlled scientific studies. We have reported the ideas in this book simply because there is some evidence that they have worked for some people. In doing this, we have attempted to separate fact from fiction and to give special attention to health tips which have been confirmed by scientific research. We have attempted, wherever possible, to verify the accuracy of information reported in this book. Nevertheless, since these are only reports of the research or ideas of other people, we cannot guarantee their safety or effectiveness.

Because of the possibility of errors in reporting the research of others, and because medical science is such a rapidly expanding field with new developments reported each day, we ask that you consult carefully with your own physician before trying any of the health tips listed in this book.

The health tips reported in this book are not guaranteed to succeed with everyone. As we wrote this book, we realized that we could not pass judgment on the effectiveness of most health tips that we discovered. Some of these tips may work for you but not for other people. Some may work for others but not for you.

It can be dangerous to rely on self-treatment or home remedies and neglect proven medical treatments, such as surgery in cases of cancer. Encyclopedia of Natural Health Secrets and Cures includes standard medical treatments as well as some natural remedies. Medical treatment shouldn't be ignored, but natural prevention or treatment may help, too. A good physician is the best judge of what sort of medical treatment may be needed for certain diseases. It's good to choose a doctor who is open-minded about safe, natural methods of prevention and treatment.

Good luck as you strive for a naturally healthier life. We believe these tips will help.

Allergy Relief

•• "Indoor air pollution", especially in tightly sealed, super-insulated houses, can cause severe allergic reactions. Irritability, headaches, forgetfulness, sore throats, nausea and tiredness have all been connected to vapors, dust or airborne particles found within our homes. If indoor air pollution is a problem, the following tips may help:

> Ban smoking in your house. Smoking increases your exposure to benzene by ten times, according to <u>Medical</u> <u>Update</u> (10:9). Even non-smokers who live in the same house as a smoker are at an increased risk. They will receive 50% more benzene exposure than the average person. Benzene is known to be an allergen (an allergy causing substance) and a carcinogen (a cancer-causing agent) that can cause leukemia.

> Chloroform has been found in four to five times greater amounts inside homes than in the outside air. <u>The</u> <u>International</u> <u>Medical</u> <u>Tribune</u> suggests that showers are the sources of chloroform. When chlorine is added to the water supply, it reacts with organic molecules in the water to form chloroform. This cholorform is released into the household air when hot water is sprayed from the shower. Using a bathroom fan that blows warm air outside can reduce high levels

of chloroform in the house.

> A leaky gas stove can cause headaches and other health problems as high levels of nitrogen dioxide build up in the house. If you have a gas oven, have it inspected annually. Have the oven and each burner properly vented, and open your windows often to air out the house.

> Other sources of heat can also produce unwanted gases. Wood-burning stoves, fireplaces, kerosene heaters or oil-burning heaters all need to be properly vented to avoid a dangerous buildup of fumes.

> Check for radon gas or asbestos in your home because they can cause severe allergic reactions in sensitive people. Radon gas is a radioactive byproduct of uranium that can seep into a house through basements, concrete floors, floor drains, cracks, or through your water if you have a private well. Asbestos is a known cancer-causing agent that was used in insulation, floorboard, wallboard, and plaster in homes and buildings constructed before 1972.

. > To avoid chemical buildup within the home, allergy prone people can open their windows and screened doors more often. However, many allergens from plants come airborne into homes. People who are sensitive to pollen will have to weigh the consequences of having more pollen in their homes (caused by open windows) to having high levels of chemicals that can accumulate in a completely closed house.

> Hang dry-cleaned clothes outdoors for a couple of hours before bringing them inside. One of the most common dry-cleaning solvents, tetrachloroethylene, can remain in a house for up to two weeks after clothes are returned from the dry cleaner.

> Formaldehyde is often contained in building materials like pressed wood paneling. People living in a brand-new home or a mobile home may come in contact with formaldehyde which can cause skin, nose, eye and throat problems as well as headaches and nausea. Formaldehyde fumes from improperly cured foam insulation have been a problem in the past, but formaldehyde-based insulation is no longer used. However, people with older homes may still have problems.

> Avoid using aerosol sprays of any kind. In an enclosed space, like your house, aerosol sprays can release high amounts of dangerous chemicals.

> Keep cleaning supplies, bleach, paint, paint removers, oven cleaners, floor polish, and pesticides outside if possible. A common chemical found in many of these products is methylene

chloride, which is suspected by the Consumer Federation of America to be a cause of diabetes and nervous disorders. It is also suspected of being a carcinogen because it has produced cancerous tumors in laboratory animals.

•• Avoid sulfites. These are chemical preservatives sometimes used in processed foods. Sulfites can cause severe reactions in sensitive people and asthmatics including wheezing, hives, dizziness and bronchial constriction that could lead to death. After 13 deaths due to sulfites and over 800 complaints that were submitted to the Food and Drug Administration (FDA), banned the used of sulfites on fresh fruits and vegetables to be sold or served raw to consumers. New labelling laws for meat, poultry and alcoholic beverages should make it easier for sulfite-sensitive people.

To eliminate sulfites, avoid foods containing sulfur dioxide, sodium sulfite, sodium and potassium bisulfite, and sodium and potassium metabisulfite. According to the FDA, sulfites are most commonly used in:

> alcoholic beverages

> baked goods including cookies, crackers, pie crusts, pizza crust, and flour tortillas

> condiments like horseradish, relishes, pickles, olives, and salad dressing mixes

> brown, raw, powdered, or white sugar from sugar beets

> fish including canned clams, shrimp, frozen lobster, scallops and dried cod

> processed fruits like juices, dried fruit, and maraschino cherries

> processed vegetables

> puddings, gelatins and fillings

> grain products and pasta including cornstarch, spinach pasta, hominy, breading and noodle/rice mixes

> jams and jellies

> canned and dried soup

> sauces including corn syrup, maple syrup, pancake syrup and molasses

> instant tea

> some prescription and non-prescription drugs

•• Allergies to cosmetic preparations can be reduced or avoided if you follow these tips:

> Start using new products just one at a time. By introducing only one new product at a time, you will be able to determine your body's reaction to it alone. However, if you start using two or more products at the same time, it will be difficult to pinpoint exactly which one is causing your reaction.

> Never put a new product directly on your face. Test it on your forearm or on the inside of your elbow. Place the product there twice a day for a minimum of four days. If a rash or other adverse reaction occurs, do NOT use that product. Even if your test turns out negative, be careful to watch for any unusual reactions that could occur after you start using any new product.

> Notice any change in reactions to your regular cosmetics. Manufacturers often reformulate their products without notice. A new ingredient in a familiar product could bother you.

> According to a study by the North American Contact Dermatitis Group, fragrances cause most of the allergic reactions to cosmetics. If you are allergic to fragrances, use products that are unscented or fragrance-free. Use caution. Many products that are unscented actually have several fragrances that are combined to produce an unscented final product so you should check the ingredient list for fragrances.

> Limit your use of skin-care products (like creams and lotions), hair-care products (like coloring, perms, or shampoo) and facial make-up (like foundation and blush). These are the top three product categories that have been discovered by the North American Contact Dermatitis Group

study to cause allergies.

> Always read the labels of cosmetic products and avoid any substances that you know will bother you.

> Have a skin test at a beauty parlor several days before getting your hair colored or permed. Severe skin problems, swelling of the throat, and death can occur as a strong reaction to these hair products.

> Always use clean applicators, like sponges, brushes and puffs, for all your cosmetics. Dirty applicators can cause allergic reactions. Never use someone else's applicator, and do not allow anyone to use yours.

Alzheimer's Disease

Alzheimer's disease is difficult to diagnose. Furthermore, as memory degenerates and confusion takes over, care of an Alzheimer's patient may become difficult. It is estimated that over 2.5 million Americans suffer from some form of this disease.

•• There is no proven cure, but avoiding smoking may help to prevent it according to a recent Harvard University study by Stuart Shalat.

•• New research by doctors at Harvard Medical

School shows that Alzheimer's may be an inherited disorder (Science 2/24/87). A defective gene has been found on the same chromosome on which a different defect causes Down's Syndrome. Doctors hope that this discovery will aid in finding the cause of Alzheimer's and how it can be treated or prevented.

•• A preliminary study by researchers at the University of California at San Francisco indicates that blows to the head early in life may be a cause of memory loss and other Alzheimer's symptoms later in life. The report in the Journal of the American Medical Association (JAMA 257,17:2289) noted that two out of three studies showed a direct relationship between head trauma and the development of Alzheimer's.

•• Columbia University's Health and Nutrition Newsletter (3:2) suggests several ways to help cope with an Alzheimer's victim:

> If Alzheimer's is suspected, be sure to have the person examined by a doctor. Several serious but treatable diseases can cause the memory loss and confusion that are often attributed to Alzheimer's disease. Strokes, brain tumors, prescription drugs, heart attacks, chronic insomnia, heart failure, irregular heart rhythms, kidney or liver failure, high or low blood sugar, thyroid

problems, lung disease, dehydration and nutritional deficiencies can cause symptoms similar to Alzheimer's disease.

> Keep the surroundings familiar to the patient. Don't move furniture or change the home in a drastic way. Try to provide a consistent environment for the person. Keep an Alzheimer's patient in his community since traveling can be very disconcerting.

> Don't allow the person to wander away from home. Alzheimer's victims should wear an I.D. bracelet or chain that identifies them as an Alzheimer's patient and gives their home address and phone number.

> If just minor memory loss has occurred, help the person by making lists and setting alarm clocks for times to take drugs or eat. As the memory loss progresses, you may need to take the person to the bathroom at certain intervals since he may not remember to go on his own. A high-fiber diet and drinking lots of fluids should help maintain regularity.

> Encourage the person to eat a healthful, balanced diet and do not allow alcoholic beverages. Alzheimer's victims may reject some important foods, but try to creatively provide good nutrition for them. Research has linked some nutritional deficiencies to Alzheimer's disease, but

conclusive evidence is not yet available. Therefore, maintaining a well-balanced diet is extremely important.

> You may need to remind the person to brush his teeth. If the patient is unable to or refuses to brush his teeth, someone should help him or the teeth will quickly deteriorate.

> Help reinforce familiar information. Names of family members may be forgotten, so keep labeled family pictures around to reinforce the names. Labeling simple tasks that are now difficult may also help the patient. For example, tape "OFF" and "ON" onto light switches.

> Keep new information simple and fresh. Don't expect the person to remember new information. Tell him about it just before the event or activity. Otherwise, it could be forgotten.

> Allow simple decisions. Even though people with Alzheimer's may have a difficult time making decisions, be sure to encourage them. It is easier for them to choose between two options rather than to make an open-ended decision. For example, "Would you like to read or would you like to go for a walk?", is better than "What would you like to do?"

> Concentrate on the skills they have rather than the skills they have lost. Encourage them to

do the things they can do and enjoy doing.

> Provide lots of touching and obvious love. Although Alzheimer patients don't realize exactly what has happened, they do sense frustration and feel that "something" is wrong. Hugging and touching provide reassurance and aid relaxation.

> Try to keep Alzheimer's victims in good mental spirits and encourage suitable exercise so the body stays as healthy as possible. Walking with or without a walker is great exercise. Even rocking in a chair exercises some muscles and helps to keep blood flowing.

Appendicitis

Research at the University of Southampton in England shows that eating tomatoes and green vegetables may reduce your chances of having appendicitis. The researchers believe that special fiber in these foods could help prevent inflammation of the appendix (<u>British</u> <u>Medical</u> <u>Journal</u>).

If you suspect appendicitis because of severe abdominal pain, nausea or fever, go to an emergency room or a doctor as soon as possible. Do not drink any fluids or take any drugs or laxatives since the doctor may need to operate to remove the swollen appendix. Food, drinks or laxatives will cause movement in the intestines, which could result in the appendix rupturing.

Arthritis

•• A recent study at Vanderbilt University Medical School showed that people with fewer than eight years of formal education had more severe rheumatoid arthritis than people with more education. The researchers believe that less-educated people are more likely to die from rheumatoid arthritis than people with at least two years of college because the less-educated do not know how to take care of their illness.

•• Royal Jelly, made from the substance that honey bees produce for the queen bee, appears to help some arthritis sufferers but not all, says Dr. Gary Meyerson of Northside Hospital in Atlanta. Royal Jelly is a white food substance that contains pantothenic acid (vitamin B5), which may also be helpful in treating rheumatoid arthritis. Dr. Meyerson believes that more research should be done on Royal Jelly because it has "great potential."

•• Aspirin is still the best single medicine to help relieve the pain and swelling of arthritis.

However, to keep the pain under control, high doses of aspirin are often required. Be sure to visit your doctor and remain under his regular care even if he advises a non-prescription product like aspirin. High doses of aspirin can reduce the ability of blood to clot and lead to ringing in the ears and stomach irritation.

Buffered aspirin, coated aspirin or time-released aspirin may cause fewer side effects than regular aspirin, especially when taken in high doses. Be sure you buy an aspirin product and not acetaminophen. Acetaminophen is the active ingredient in Tylenol®, Datril®, Panadol®, Phenaphen®, and Anacin-3®. It is a good pain-reliever but it will not control the swelling of arthritis as aspirin will. Like aspirin, ibuprofen products (including Advil®, Nuprin®, Medipren®, Motrin®, Rufen®, Trendar® and Haltran®) can control both the pain and swelling of arthritis.

•• Research has now linked one type of arthritis, rheumatoid arthritis, with an inherited defective gene and with a virus. Doctors reporting in the <u>Journal of the American Medical Association</u> (JAMA 257: 17, 2267) hope that discovering the causes of arthritis will lead to better treatment and an eventual cure.

•• Major stressful events have been associated

with the development of rheumatoid arthritis according to research by Dr. Fred Kantrowitz of the Harvard Medical School. Doctors are not certain whether a stress-filled event actually causes the arthritis or just makes it noticeable. Studies have shown that nearly 10% of women and 25% of children who develop rheumatoid arthritis have experienced a traumatic event.

•• Learning to use your body properly can help reduce the pain and swelling of arthritic joints. Here are some sensible tips from the Arthritis Foundation that can reduce the strain on your joints:

> Be efficient and save steps when using your joints. When walking, use the shortest possible route. Get extra phones and use them throughout the house or use a cordless phone that you can move with you. Apply for a handicapped-parking permit. Many people with moderate to severe arthritis are eligible for a handicapped permit.

> Use mechanical devices that will help reduce use of your joints. For example, a remote-control TV, stereo and VCR, including volume control, can save many steps. Put lights on timers to help eliminate the need to turn them off and on. A whistle switcher or sound-activated control could save steps. A push-button phone programmed for

your most frequently used numbers can be helpful.

> Make your car as easy to use as possible. Use automatic transmission, power windows, power brakes, power door locks, automatic trunk release and any other options that will reduce your need to move.

> Make living within your home as convenient as possible. Try to live on just one level of your house to avoid climbing stairs. Be creative with where you put things that you use frequently. Don't just keep them where you and others have traditionally placed them. For example, you may decide to put your washer and dryer near your bedroom to save steps. Develop "work centers" so that everything you need for a task is within easy grasp.

> Reduce the amount of bending you need to do. Keep everyday utensils on the counter or stove top so you don't have to bend down to get them. Even though it may not look as tidy, your kitchen will be easier for you to use and enjoy. Store your most-used items at your body level. Place a chair or stool in front of sinks so you can sit at the sink rather than bending over it.

> Use a bench in your bathtub or shower so you can sit while showering. Install grab bars in your shower or over your tub. To prevent slipping,

use adhesive rubber strips on the tub or shower floor rather than rubber mats.

> Make your home safe. Put adhesive rubber strips on stairs. Eliminate scatter rugs or tape them to the floor. Put wires and cables behind furniture where they will be out of the way. Make sure the inside and the outside of your home are well-lit so you can see to avoid any obstacles.

> Use comfortable and practical furniture throughout your house and patio. Firm, supportive chairs will be better for you than plush chairs or sofas that are difficult to get in and out of. You may consider getting a lift-chair that helps raise you to a standing position.

> Choose your clothes carefully. Avoid shirts or dresses that fasten up the back. Women can wear bras with a front closure rather than hooks at the back. Use velcro for fasteners. Wear clothes that will keep you comfortable. Buy shoes that are supportive and fit well. For wearing around the house, tennis shoes might be the most comfortable choice. Shoes do not have to be expensive to be well-made and supportive. Do not wear high heels, or wear only heels that are less than one inch high.

> Reduce or eliminate lifting. Push or slide objects or ask someone else to move large objects. Use as much of your body as possible when

pushing so there is less strain on an individual joint. For example, don't use your fingers when you can push with your entire hand and perhaps your shoulder. When it is necessary to lift something, use proper lifting techniques. Always use the legs to do the lifting, and bend from the knees, not from the waist. Concentrate on using your thigh muscles (at the top of your legs) rather than your back muscles. Never twist while lifting. Keep the object you are lifting as close to your body as possible. Even when you are lifting or carrying everyday items, make them as light as you can. Ladies should consider using a smaller purse, for example. Store food in plastic bags or aluminum foil rather than in heavy cooking dishes.

> Within your home, use a cart to help move items from room to room. A cart can be used to help carry dishes, laundry, cleaning supplies and food.

> When serving large numbers of people, use a "buffet-style" set-up so the guests can help themselves to plates, food and drinks. Using one table will save you many steps back and forth to the kitchen.

> Use an electric can opener and an under-the-counter jar opener. The jar opener will allow you to open all sizes of jars without harming your

joints.

> If you need a walker, get one with wheels and auto-stops on it because you can roll it without having to lift it. If you use a cane, an adjustable model allowing you to change the height for each situation might be best. The cane should be used on the side of the body that is least affected by the arthritis.

> Using a typewriter rather than writing with a pen or pencil may be helpful. Many people find that typing doesn't bother their joints as much as holding onto a pen or pencil. Consider using a "light touch" typewriter or home computer. When writing, use a felt-tip pen instead of a ball point pen since the felt-tip pen doesn't require as much pressure.

> If grasping small items like pens and table utensils is difficult, try placing a soft foam curler around the item. This will make it larger and softer to hold. Keep a "jar opener" pad in your purse or pocket. You can use the non-slip rubber pad to open doorknobs or other objects even when you are away from home.

> If getting money out of pay-telephones or vending machines is difficult, try using the eraser-end of a pencil to slide the coin out of the slot and into your hand.

> Keep as active as possible. To avoid stiffness, try not to remain in the same position for more than 20 minutes. Maintain good posture when sitting and standing. A ten-year study in The Lancet showed that moderate activity was better than bed rest for sufferers of rheumatoid arthritis.

> Balance your activity with adequate rest. Interrupt long spells of activity with short breaks. Try to get 10 to 12 hours of sleep per night. Most arthritis sufferers seem to need much sleep.

> Plan your schedule around the times your arthritis is most painful. For example, many people find that they're able to enjoy certain activities more in the afternoon than in the morning because most of their joint stiffness has subsided then.

Asthma

•• When exercising, asthmatics should use their legs and limit the use of their arms. According to a study in The New England Journal of Medicine (314:23,1485), even people who have severe asthmatic bouts when brushing their hair or using their arms can tolerate moderate exercise with their legs. Any upper-body movement with the arms unsupported, puts additional strain on the muscles used for breathing. Upper-body movement should be limited in asthmatics, but thorough workouts of the legs can help the asthmatic stay in shape.

•• Avoid sulfites, chemicals used to preserve processed foods. Sulfites can cause severe asthmatic reactions, including wheezing, hives, dizziness and bronchial constriction that could lead to death. See our section on **Allergies** for a complete list of sulfites and processed foods which sometimes contain sulfites.

•• Avoid inactivity. Prolonged time lying down can allow mucus to accumulate in the lungs.

•• Do not participate in woodworking. Dusts and fumes from freshly cut wood such as pine, birch, mahogany and red cedar are known to contribute to asthma attacks. Keep any woodworking activities away from the home of an asthmatic.

•• Avoid living or working near industrial or electric utility smokestacks which produce sulfur dioxide. The Environmental Protection Agency (EPA) says that sulfur dioxide from such smokestacks can make breathing more difficult for asthmatics — especially asthmatics who exercise outdoors. Many areas in the northeastern and southeastern United States should be avoided because these areas have high levels of sulfur dioxide emissions which are converted in the atmosphere to sulphuric acid. The sulphuric acid often returns to earth in precipitation known as "acid rain."

•• Keep emotionally healthy. Recent studies in the Journal of the American Medical Association (JAMA 254: 1193-8) show that an inordinate number of depressed asthmatics are dying. Dr. Robert Strunk of the National Jewish Center for Immunology and Respiratory Medicine in Denver conducted research which discovered that emotional stability, especially in an asthmatic child, can affect the severeness of the attacks. He believes that some children with severe asthma actually "will themselves to death" because of the agonizing frustration of their disease.

Back Pain

•• Two days of bed rest are enough for relieving back problems due to muscle pain, according to research by Richard Deyo, M.D., (The New England Journal of Medicine 315: 1064). The study compared people with back pain who rested for two days with those who rested for seven. Follow-up examinations at three weeks and at three months showed no difference between the two groups. The doctors concluded that two days of bed rest are sufficient.

•• To avoid back pain, the American Academy of Orthopedic Surgeons recommends:

> Never use your back muscles to lift. Bend at the knees and use your thigh muscles (at the top of your legs) to lift and properly support heavy weight.

> Sleep on a firm, supportive mattress.

> Maintain your "ideal" weight.

> Exercise your whole body, including your back muscles, regularly.

Bedwetting

According to the American Journal of Diseases of Children (140:260), many older children who wet the bed suffer from constipation. Doctors report that the additional pressure on the bladder from a full colon can cause bedwetting. Adding fiber to the child's diet and having periodic rectal exams to determine the cause of constipation may help to solve bedwetting problems.

Bites By Insects

•• Many quick and easy methods are available to relieve the itch and sting of insect bites.

> Wash the bite with soap and water to remove some of the venom and reduce the pain.

> Place ice directly on the bite.

> Wash the bite with rubbing alcohol or vinegar.

> Apply cream or lotion containing hydrocortisone.

> If you are outdoors try applying mud or the sap from a jewelweed plant.

> Some people recommend applying common meat tenderizers, but a recent study in The Journal of the American Academy of Dermatology tested this remedy on fire-ant stings. They discovered that the meat tenderizer has "no value" in treating these stings. However, the researchers said that the papain in meat tenderizer may relieve the pain of some other insect bites.

•• The best way to prevent insect bites is to protect yourself from being bitten. When going outdoors:

> Use an insect repellent containing N, N-diethyl-meta-toluamide or DEET only after considering its risks. Studies show that DEET is absorbed through the skin of animals and causes injury to the brain.

> Use a "rub-on" rather than a spray repellent.

> Place the repellent on any exposed skin,

especially remembering the neck, ankles and wrists.

> If you go swimming or get wet with perspiration, re-apply the repellent.

> In The Vitamin Bible, Dr. Earl Mindell recommends taking thiamine (vitamin B1) supplements to help your skin develop a "natural" repellent. Mindell suggests taking 100 mg. of thiamine three times daily to create an odor "at the level of your skin" that insects do not like.

> When outdoors, wear long pants, a long-sleeved shirt and a hat, so as little skin as possible is exposed.

> If a bite or sting causes unusual swelling or a severe reaction, get the person to the hospital immediately, since many people are seriously allergic to bites.

Blood Pressure — High

•• Calcium supplements may help to lower cases of high blood pressure. According to new research published in Drug Therapy (16,11:63), many people do not get enough calcium. Inadequate calcium can lead to high blood pressure. Another study indicates that people with high blood pressure consume 20 to 25% less calcium than people who don't have high blood pressure. Since taking calcium supplements or increasing the amount of calcium in the diet has few harmful side effects, extra calcium could be part of a blood pressure reducing therapy. However, do not stop taking blood pressure medication unless so advised by your doctor.

Dairy products, salmon, sardines and leafy green vegetables are the best natural sources of calcium. Calcium supplementation should be avoided by people who have kidney stones or by those with high blood-levels of calcium which make them more inclined to develop kidney stones.

•• Many studies indicate that various types of exercise help control high blood pressure. Exercise which increases the strength of the heart may help to prevent or lower high blood pressure. But don't exercise and drink alcoholic beverages. A new study at the Medical College of Wisconsin revealed that drinking just two alcoholic drinks per day can undo all of the blood-pressure reducing effects of exercising. Excessive drinking of alcohol is a major cause of high blood pressure. Alcohol damages the liver and kidneys, causing fluid buildup in the body which makes blood pressure skyrocket.

•• High blood pressure has been associated

with higher death rates in cancer patients (<u>Journal</u> <u>of</u> <u>the</u> <u>National</u> <u>Cancer</u> <u>Institute</u> 77:1,63). The higher the blood pressure, the more likely the patient was to die from the cancer, the researchers discovered.

•• Cancer itself may cause high blood pressure. Several studies have linked high blood pressure and cancer, but a new Canadian study shows that cancer may cause high blood pressure. Until now, many researchers believed that high blood pressure increased one's risk of developing cancer. But, the study in the medical journal <u>Cancer</u> (59:7,1386) revealed that blood pressure increased due to the cancer, rather than causing the cancer.

•• Reducing salt consumption is high on the priority list for effective treatment of high blood pressure. Table salt and salty products can be easy to avoid, but it is the "hidden salt" that often has consumers stumped. The Food and Drug Administration (FDA) is now requiring soft-drink manufacturers to list the sodium content of their drinks on the bottles or cans. Sodium-free drinks will have to contain less than 5 milligrams (mg.) of sodium per 12 oz. can. "Very low sodium" will be less than 35 mg. per can and "low sodium" can be placed on cans containing 140 mg. of sodium or less. Most processed foods like soup, TV-dinners, canned or frozen fruit and vegetables contain high quantities of salt.

•• A little creativity in your cooking can help add "spice" to your food while lowering the salt content. You do not have to sacrifice flavor when you cut down on sodium if you follow these suggestions from <u>Prevention</u> magazine:

> In baking cakes, cookies, pies and puddings use extracts instead of salt and reduce the sugar.

> Learn about the many natural herbs and spices that are available. You may decide to grow your own or to experiment with store-bought herbs.

> Enjoy Mexican, Cajun, spicy oriental and Tex-Mex foods. The strong spices give flavor without adding salt.

> To spice chicken dishes, add fruit such as mandarin oranges or pineapples.

> Marinate chicken, fish, beef or poultry in orange juice or lemon juice. Add a mustard or honey glaze.

> Marinate meat in wine or add wine to sauces or soups. If you thoroughly cook the dish, the alcohol will evaporate but the flavor will be enhanced.

> Add unsalted nuts, sunflower seeds, sesame seeds or water chestnuts to any meat dish or salad.

> Just a little green pepper, parsley, paprika or

red pepper can add a lot of flavor to a meal.

> Instead of adding pork fat or lard to baked beans, try adding a small amount of beer.

Bronchitis

•• Don't smoke. When you quit smoking you decrease the risk of developing bronchitis or other lung diseases. If you have already developed bronchitis, continued smoking will increase the severity of the disease.

•• Don't live or work in a smoke-filled environment. According to the U.S. Surgeon General, Dr. C. Everett Koop, children under the age of two who live with parents who smoke have an increased risk of developing bronchitis or pneumonia.

•• Avoid all types of air pollution. Avoid exposure to any airborne substance that is a known irritant including:

> chlorine fumes
> hydrogen sulfide fumes
> sulfur dioxide fumes
> bromine fumes
> ammonia fumes
> air pollutants
> mineral or vegetable dusts

> dusts from woodworking or baking
> aerosol sprays

•• When traveling, avoid large cities or areas known to have high air pollution. Make reservations at hotels that offer "no smoking" accommodations. Use air conditioning during the warm months so you will not have to open windows and bring in unclean air.

•• In a plane, sit as far away from the smoking section as possible. Travel only in pressurized planes. Some commuter flights are not pressurized and could make your breathing very difficult.

•• For a pollution-free vacation, consider a cruise. The air quality is excellent and a doctor is usually available if any problems arise.

•• Don't travel to areas with high elevation. The higher the elevation the more difficult it will be for you to breathe.

•• When driving in considerable traffic, try traveling before rush hour or after dusk when the air quality is at its best. Use the air-conditioning in your car and never open your windows in polluted areas.

•• Drink at least eight glasses of water each day. Water will help keep the throat clear by diluting the mucus and keep it moist. Breathing the steam from hot liquids, like chicken soup, will also help keep the throat and breathing passages clear.

•• Inhaling steam from a vaporizer, kettle or shower may be helpful.

•• Do not use cough suppressants except in extreme cases where the cough is not allowing you to get adequate sleep. In bronchitis it is important that any loose phlegm be coughed up. Do not try to stop the coughing.

•• Place the head lower than the chest to help in breathing. Lying on your stomach with your head hanging down off the side of the bed may provide easier breathing.

•• Since infections can be extremely dangerous to a person with bronchitis:

> Be sure to get all vaccines prescribed by your doctor.

> Get plenty of rest.

> Eat a well-balanced diet.

> Avoid unnecessary exposure to infections.

Cancer

•• Regular exercise is important for a person undergoing cancer treatment, indicates <u>Physician and Sportsmedicine</u> (14,10:125). Even though cancer patients need plenty of rest, regular exercise helps them keep a positive attitude, which is important in their treatment. Exercise also helps reduce the length of nausea experienced after chemotherapy, the study reports.

•• Vitamin E may help chemotherapy patients keep more of their hair, according to new preliminary research by Dr. Lee Wood of California. In patients who would be undergoing treatment with doxorubicin, Dr. Wood gave them 1600 International Units (IU's) of vitamin E daily for several days. When they started chemotherapy with doxorubicin, only 30% of the people taking vitamin E had significant hair loss. Usually 100% of people taking doxorubicin lose their hair!

•• Foods rich in vitamin E or beta-carotene may help defend you against lung cancer, reports The New England Journal of Medicine. People with low blood levels of vitamin E were 2 1/2 times more likely to get lung cancer. Low levels of beta-carotene could increase your chances of getting lung cancer by four times, concludes a study from Johns Hopkins University. Another study by the State University of New York at Buffalo confirmed the link between beta-carotene and lung cancer. Yet the difference between the diet of lung cancer patients and healthy individuals was the amount of beta-carotene found in one carrot, the study reported in the American Journal of Epidemiology (125:3,351). Whole grains and nuts contain high amounts of vitamin E. Yellow or orange vegetables or fruits, like carrots, are particularly good sources of beta-carotene, which the healthy body converts to vitamin A.

•• Cleaning supplies, bleach, paint, paint removers, oven cleaners, floor polish, and pesticides should be kept away from living areas if possible. Many of these products contain methylene chloride, a suspected carcinogen that has produced cancerous tumors in laboratory animals, reports the Consumer Federation of America.

•• Small quantities of jalapeno and cayenne peppers may help reduce the risk of cancer, according to a report from Dr. Peter M. Gannett of the Eppley Institute. Hot peppers contain capsaicin, which is changed into a chemical that absorbs free radicals in the liver. Free radicals are thought to cause cancer, so capsaicin may help reduce cancer. However, since large amounts of capsaicin can cause changes in blood pressure, brain damage and stomach ulcers, only small amounts of peppers are recommended.

•• Don't smoke. As well as increasing your chances of getting lung cancer, smoking affects other types of cancers. Smoking increases a person's exposure to benzene by ten times according to Medical Update (10:9). Benzene is known to be a cancer-causing agent (a carcinogen) that can cause leukemia. Even non-smokers who live in the same house as a smoker are at an increased risk. They will receive 50% more benzene exposure than the average person. To avoid excessive benzene exposure, do not live or work in a smoke-filled environment.

In 1985, 60 non-smoking Canadian spouses died from lung cancer that is believed to have been caused by their spouses' smoking (Canadian Medical Association Journal), but not necessarily related to benzene levels.

Parents who smoke should know that their children under the age of two have an increased risk of developing pneumonia or bronchitis, according to the U.S. Surgeon General, Dr. C. Everett Koop.

Another recent study at the University of California found that smokers were twice as likely to develop cancer of the colon as were non-smokers. (Cancer 58:3,784).

People who are diagnosed as having any type of cancer need to give up smoking. A new study shows that nicotine actually speeds up cancer's growth in the body. Dr. Gesina Longenecker of the

University of Southern Alabama School of Medicine, who made the discovery, recommends that all cancer patients quit smoking as soon as possible to slow down their cancer's development. Dr. Longenecker encourages cancer patients to quit smoking "cold turkey" rather than using a prescription gum called Nicorette® because the chewing gum also contains the dangerous nicotine which speeds up the cancer.

•• Check for radon gas. According to the Environmental Protection Agency (EPA), high levels of radon gas in homes may be the second leading cause of lung cancer. Radon gas is a radioactive byproduct of uranium that has been found in over 30 states. It is a gas that can seep into a house through concrete floors, floor drains, cracks, or through your water if you have a private well. To check your home's radon gas level, call the local EPA or health department. To reduce exposure to radon gas keep your house well-ventilated and limit the amount of time you spend in the basement where the gas levels are usually higher. Do not allow smoking in your home since radon can attach to the small particles of tobacco smoke where they can be inhaled directly into the body and trapped in the lungs.

•• Consider where you live. Like radon gas,

living close to large chemical plants, polluted water, waste disposal areas, certain industries or natural deposits of minerals could increase your risk of getting cancer. Learn more about your neighborhood. If the risk of getting cancer is increased, you may want to relocate.

•• Limit or eliminate the use of pesticides inside the home. A recent study in the <u>Journal</u> <u>of</u> <u>the</u> <u>National</u> <u>Cancer</u> <u>Institute</u> showed that children in homes where indoor pesticides were used once a week were 3.8 times more likely to develop leukemia. If pesticides were also used regularly in the garden or elsewhere outside, the children's risk of developing cancer increased to 6.5 times compared to unexposed children.

•• Think about changing your job. The American Institute for Cancer Research (AICR) estimates "that one to four percent of all cancers are work-related." For example, bladder cancer occurs more often in people employed as dye workers or in other jobs in the chemical industry. Your job can cause cancer in your body up to 50 years after the time you were exposed. So, even if you feel well, you may want to consider changing your job or profession. Cancer can be caused by work-place exposure to:

> arsenic

> benzene
> chromium
> coal, tar or soot
> dyes
> ethers
> iron oxide
> leather dust
> petroleum
> vinyl chloride
> x-rays

•• Use certified pure spring water for drinking and cooking, instead of regular tap water. The Environmental Protection Agency (EPA) has identified and set standards on eight carcinogens (known cancer-causing substances) that are commonly found in drinking water. However, the EPA acknowledges that not all city or county water systems meet these standards. Also, another EPA report by Michael Alavanja, Inge Goldstein and Mervyn Susser showed a correlation between drinking chlorinated water and having a higher risk of developing cancer. If you cannot afford spring water, trying boiling all water before using it. If possible, let the water sit out in an uncovered container for at least 24 hours so that chlorine will be released into the air and the water will be a little safer to use.

•• Check for asbestos. Asbestos is a known

cancer-causing agent. It was used in insulation, floorboard, wallboard, and plaster in homes and buildings constructed before 1972. As long as the asbestos is not disintegrating or flaky, it can be carefully covered and left intact. However, if any asbestos-containing material starts to disintegrate, a professional should be called in to remove it. If you have questions about asbestos in your home, office or school you can call your local Environmental Protection Agency (EPA) office or 1-800-835-6700.

•• According to Time's <u>Symptoms</u> <u>and</u> <u>Illnesses</u>, lung cancer is often caused by exposure to:

> asbestos
> chromium
> nickel
> iron
> petroleum oil mists
> cigarette, cigar and pipe smoke
> isopropyl oil
> coal tar fumes
> air pollution
> radioactive substances

•• Children who are exposed to the magnetic fields from overhead power lines are at an increased risk of developing brain cancer or leukemia according to a new study by the New York Power Lines Project. The researchers believe that power lines could be responsible for up to 15% of all childhood cancers. Unfortunately, rarely encountered long distance high-voltage wires are not believed to be the problem. Common overhead high-current wires that link individual homes to the local power supply seem to be the most dangerous.

•• Men should consume plenty of selenium according to studies conducted in The Netherlands (American Journal of Epidemiology 125,1:12). In the study at Erasumus University in Rotterdam, men with cancers were found to have "significantly lower" levels of selenium in their blood than men without cancer. However, there was no difference in the blood levels of selenium in women. Other population studies have shown that areas of the country where selenium is high in food or in the water have low rates of cancer. It is recommended that adults consume 50 to 200 micrograms of selenium daily. Natural selenium sources include liver and other organ meats, seafood, eggs, onions, meat, poultry, grains, cereals, dairy products and vegetables. Selenium is an antioxidant which may help to protect against cancer as it fights free radicals in the body.

•• Reduce or eliminate tea from your diet. According to a study in Hawaii, men who drank tea more than once a day had a four times greater risk of developing rectal cancer than men who "almost never" drank tea. (British Journal of Cancer 54:5,677). The test included tea made from black tea leaves which had been brewed to make tea. It did not differentiate between hot or iced tea. Other medical studies have made a connection between drinking tea and developing kidney, pancreas or bladder cancer.

•• Rectal cancer may be influenced by the level of cholesterol in the blood. According to Swedish research published in The New England Journal of Medicine (315:26,1629), high levels of cholesterol increased the risk of developing rectal cancer by 1.65 times over average levels. Another study in the same issue of the journal reports that people with high levels of cholesterol were twice as likely to develop colon polyps as people with low cholesterol levels.

All men over 50 years of age should have a yearly rectal exam for signs of prostate and other cancers since the incidence is highest in this age group.

•• Eliminate or consume only small amounts of food that is smoked, salt-cured, pickled, cooked over wood or charcoal, treated with nitrites, or processed. According to the <u>Nutrition</u> <u>and</u> <u>Health</u> newsletter from Columbia University (8:6), these foods increase the risk of developing stomach or esophageal cancer. Certain sausages, ham and fish readily absorb the tars from smoke or charcoal. These tars contain substances which are known to cause cancers. People should also be especially careful when traveling in China or Japan because pickled and salt-cured foods are very common there.

•• Some foods are naturally high in nitrates including raw beets, cauliflower, broccoli and cabbage. Raw spinach, lettuce, pumpkin and kosher salami are high in nitrites.

•• See the doctor if you experience prolonged stomach irritation like heartburn, nausea, bloating, loss of appetite, belching or mild pain because these could be the first signs of stomach or esophageal cancer.

•• To further reduce your risk of cancer, the American Institute for Cancer Research (AICR) recommends:

> Eat less than four ounces total of salt-cured, nitrite-cured, smoked, processed meats or charcoal-broiled foods per week.

> When eating salt-cured, nitrite-cured,

smoked or charcoal-broiled foods, also eat foods rich in vitamin C. Vitamin C is an antioxidant that may help reduce the effect of the nitrosamines in the body.

> Wrap meat, fish or poultry in aluminum foil before grilling it on charcoal.

> Baste or marinate all foods that are going to be cooked over charcoal.

> Do not eat meat that is charred.

> Do not eat crispy bacon. Bacon cooked in a microwave contains the least amount of dangerous nitrosamines.

> Throw away animal fats and oils rather than using them in soups, gravies or cooking since some pesticides become concentrated in animal fat, the fats may be more dangerous than the meat.

•• Iron deficiency has been linked to stomach and esophageal cancers, according to Nutrition and Health (8:6). Because excess iron is NOT eliminated from the body, researchers recommend consuming iron-rich foods rather than taking iron supplements. Whole-grain products, liver, organ meats, red meat, eggs, lima beans, prunes, spinach, raw broccoli, peas, fish, soy products and raisins are all good natural sources of iron.

•• Adequate amounts of the mineral molybdenum are also important in reducing the risk of stomach and esophageal cancers, reports Nutrition and Health (8:6). Molybdenum is naturally contained in whole-grain products, dark green leafy vegetables and legumes.

•• Do not eat apples, sour cherries or peanuts that have been treated with daminozide (trade name is Alar® by Uniroyal). Daminozide, a chemical used to keep apples red, delay ripening and increase their shelf-life, is absorbed by the apple and becomes incorporated into the fruit. **Washing or peeling the apple will not remove it.** According to the Food and Drug Administration (FDA), daminozide can cause cancerous tumors of the uterus, liver, kidney, blood vessels and lungs. Some stores and large baby-food manufacturers are now refusing to carry daminozide-treated products. You can't tell by inspection which apples have been treated, so buy only from stores and companies who refuse to sell or use daminozide-treated apples. American Health (16:4) recommends eating all fresh apples raw, since cooking seems to increase daminozide's cancer-causing properties. Be especially careful of these varieties of apples that the EPA says are most often treated with daminozide:
> Stayman
> McIntosh

> Golden Delicious
> Red Delicious
> Jonathan

•• According to the Environmental Protection Agency (E.P.A.) these suggestions should help decrease your exposure to other dangerous pesticides:

> Wash all fresh fruit and vegetables in warm water. Some researchers believe that it is preferable to soak them in warm water and a 1/4 cup of vinegar for about 20 minutes, then rinse them with cool water before preparing. The EPA Journal encourages consumers to scrub all vegetables and fruits with a brush.

> Fresh produce with thin skins should be peeled including apples, carrots, cucumbers, grapes, potatoes, turnips and zucchini.

> Buy only American fruit and vegetables since pesticide standards in other countries are different.

> Grow as many of your own vegetables and fruit as possible. There are no standards for "organic" produce, and you cannot tell if dangerous chemicals have been used on produce advertised as such. If you grow your own produce with resistant varieties of crops, you will know exactly what you are eating.

> If you use pesticides, do not buy any that require you to wear protective gear. Follow the label instructions exactly when applying the pesticide, storing it, and discarding it after use.

> Do not spray on windy days. Do not chew gum, drink or smoke while using pesticides. Only spray in well-ventilated areas away from children.

•• Take steps to lower your blood pressure. In people with cancer, the higher their blood pressure, the more likely they are to die from the cancer, reports the Journal of the National Cancer Institute (77:1,63).

•• Cervical cancer can be treated effectively if it is diagnosed early. If women have an annual PAP smear, they reduce their risk of developing undetected cancer of the cervix.

•• Women who have been on oral contraceptives (the "pill") for a minimum of 12 consecutive months seem to have a lower risk of developing endometrial cancer. According to a study by the Centers for Disease Control in Atlanta, the risk of getting endometrial cancer is cut in half in some women who have used the "pill" (Journal of the American Medical Association JAMA 257:6,796). However, the researchers warn that even with the benefits of lower incidence of cancer, women who smoke should not take oral contraceptives because of the increased risk of heart and artery problems.

Women who have an increased risk of developing endometrial cancer should be sure to have a gynecological exam at least once a year. The risk of developing endometrial cancer (in the lining of the uterus or womb) increases if the woman:

> does not ovulate.
> is infertile.
> is obese.
> has diabetes.
> had a late menopause.
> had long-term estrogen therapy after menopause.

•• Women who give birth to children before age 30 decrease their risk of developing breast cancer, according to research at Emory University (The New England Journal of Medicine). The level of the hormone prolactin may be the difference. Doctors report that the level of prolactin in a woman's body falls after childbirth and nursing. Since a high level of prolactin is associated with increased risk of breast cancer, childbirth seems to be a natural way to lower cancer risk in women.

•• The risk of breast cancer is slightly higher in women who have estrogen-replacement therapy

(ERT), reports the Centers for Disease Control (CDC) in Atlanta (Journal of the American Medical Association JAMA 257,2, 209). However, they suggest that women and their doctors need to weigh the proven benefits of estrogen-replacement therapy (protection against osteoporosis and heart or artery problems) against the slightly increased risk of breast cancer. Women who have a family history of breast cancer should probably avoid estrogen-replacement therapy, the study concluded.

•• Do not drink alcohol. A recent study published in The New England Journal of Medicine (316:1169) showed that women who drank even moderate amounts of alcohol had a greater risk of developing breast cancer than women who did not drink. Alcohol consumption is also linked to liver cancer.

•• High amounts of protein in a woman's diet could increase her chances of developing breast cancer according to research by Dr. E.J. Hawrylewicz of Chicago's Mercy Hospital. The American Institute for Cancer Research (AICR) reports that Dr. Hawrylewicz discovered that "feeding laboratory animals high protein diets generally increases their susceptibility to breast cancer when they are exposed to a carcinogen."

•• The American Cancer Society now recommends that women 50 and over, even if they don't have cancer or breast problems, should have a mammogram once every year. Women between 40 and 49 should have a mammogram every second year. The first mammogram should be given when a woman is between 35 and 39 years of age. The first mammogram is used as a base line to detect any irregularities later, the Society explains. A mammogram is a special x-ray of the breast which enables doctors to detect the "earliest and most curable breast cancer". Some women are at a high risk for developing breast cancer. If you fall into one of the high risk categories listed below, you should ask your doctor or gynecologist for regular mammograms:

> if you gave birth to your first child after the age of 30.

> if you have never given birth.

> if your mother or sister has developed breast cancer.

> if you reached sexual maturity very early.

> if you have a history of cysts in your breasts.

> if you are overweight.

> if you are over 40 years of age.

•• Doctors warn that the development of skin cancer is on the rise as sun bathing has become popular. In 1982, one out of every 250 people developed skin cancer. But by the year 2000, one out of every 90 will develop it, forecasts Dr. Darrel Rigel of the New York University Medical Center. Doctors suggest that everyone, especially people who spend a lot of time outdoors in the sunshine or people who are fair-skinned, should regularly examine themselves for warning signs of skin cancer. Active sunbathers, farmers, lifeguards, outdoor construction workers and sailors need to be particularly careful. A monthly "lookover" should include the body parts that are most often exposed, like your hands, face, neck, scalp and ears. According to the <u>University of California, Berkeley Wellness Letter</u> (3:9) watch for:

> Changes in the color or size of a mole or wart.

> A sore that will not heal or is slow to heal.

> Any translucent growths on your skin. Usually this type of growth is shiny and white, pink or red in people with light-colored hair. Those with dark hair should be wary of darker, translucent growths.

> Red patches on your skin. Sometimes these will crust or itch but other times you may hardly even notice them.

> A smooth bump that is indented in the

middle.

> Any scar-like growths or spots. Usually white or yellow with a waxy surface.

•• Keep a moderate amount of a variety of fibers in your diet. A new study from Texas A & M University shows that too much "mushy" fiber may lead to colon cancer. High quantities of three types of fiber, pectin (found in fruits and root vegetables), guar (found in processed foods and ice cream) and oat bran, were found to contribute to the development of colon cancer. These mushy types of fiber help to lower cholesterol, but they slow down movement through the intestines. Harder types of dietary fiber like bran help move waste products through the intestines rapidly. With less contact with the lining of the intestines, the cancer-causing substances in the intestines seemed to be less harmful. While fiber is generally beneficial, too much of a *single type* of fiber such as psyllium mucilloid supplements should be avoided. The researchers recommend getting your fiber from a wide variety of whole grain breads, cereals, fruits and vegetables.

•• Avoid laxatives containing danthron. Danthron has been proven to cause colon and liver cancer in animals. It was contained in these common laxatives until May 1987: Modane®

(Regular, Mild, Liquid and Plus), Doxidan®, Dorbantyl®, Dorbane®, Guarsol®, Danthron tablets, Key Lax® Laxative Tablets, Docusate Calcium® with Danthron and DC® with Danthron. The Public Citizens Health Letter (3:4), a Ralph Nader newsletter, suggests that you throw away any laxatives you have which contain danthron or return them to your pharmacist for a refund. Products containing danthron have been banned in Britain and the United States but some people may still have these products in their medicine cabinets.

Child Care

•• Babies who spend more than 20 hours away from their parents each week in the first year of life may develop emotional problems later on, reports a study from Penn State University. Babies in full-time day care are at heightened risk of becoming "problem" children, says Jay Belsky, a researcher at Penn State. They could become aggressive and withdraw from others as they grow older, he warns. Belsky suggests that parents should be given adequate leave time and only work part-time until the baby is at least one year old.

Cholesterol Reduction

•• High blood cholesterol levels lead to heart disease so, your blood cholesterol level and its HDL (high-density lipoprotein) and LDL (low-density lipoprotein) fractions should be checked once a year, or every time blood is drawn (if more than once a year). According to the National Institutes of Health and the American Heart Association, people over 30 years of age should maintain cholesterol levels below 200 milligrams per deciliter of blood (mg/dL). People under 30 should strive for a cholesterol level of about 180 mg/dL.

Until recently it seemed that cholesterol levels lower than 200 mg/dL did not have any corresponding advantage of a lower risk of heart disease. However, a new study, part of the Multiple Risk Factor Intervention Trial (MRFIT) has shown that the lower the cholesterol level, the lower your risk for heart disease. Based on these results, your cholesterol level should be as low as possible, because your risk of heart disease increases when your cholesterol level increases.

•• The Wellness Letter (3:9) from the University of California at Berkeley advises that various circumstances can alter your blood cholesterol levels. For example, explains the Wellness Letter, your blood cholesterol levels are usually higher in the winter than in the summer. The position your arm is in when the blood is drawn and the competency of the laboratory that analyzes the blood sample could also alter your results.

•• Women taking estrogen for problems with menopause may produce higher levels of the beneficial HDL type of cholesterol. Of the two types of cholesterol, high levels of HDL are thought to help prevent coronary heart disease, but high levels of LDL cholesterol can be very dangerous. Harvey Gruchow, who conducted the study at the Medical College of Wisconsin, says the high HDL levels were found after 900 women had an angiogram (an X-ray of the blood vessels). The angiograms showed that women taking estrogen had much less cholesterol blockage in the arteries. This study confirms the results of earlier research from the National Institutes of Health (NIH) which concluded that the death rate from heart disease in estrogen users was 1/3 the rate of women who did not take estrogen. The NIH recommends that women should take estrogen during mid-life, and especially during menopause, to lower their risk of heart disease.

•• Vitamin E may help raise the blood levels of HDL (the good cholesterol), according to a study in the <u>American</u> <u>Journal</u> <u>of</u> <u>Clinical</u> <u>Pathology</u> (3/82).

•• The combination of a low-saturated fat, low-cholesterol diet with a prescription drug, colestipol, and large doses of a cholesterol-lowering vitamin, niacin, has been proven to reduce the blood level of cholesterol and reduce further damage to the heart and arteries in non-smoking men who had already had heart bypass surgery. Total cholesterol level dropped by 26% in those taking colestipol and niacin. However, cholesterol levels dropped only 4% in men who were on the same diet but did not receive the drug and vitamin, according to the <u>Journal</u> <u>of</u> <u>the</u> <u>American</u> <u>Medical</u> <u>Association</u> (JAMA 257:3233-40).

•• High quantities of lecithin combined with a low-saturated fat, low-cholesterol diet may help to lower cholesterol levels more than diet alone, according to Ronald K. Tompkins, M.D. (<u>American</u> <u>Journal</u> <u>of</u> <u>Surgery</u> 140:3). In Dr. Tompkin's study, each person received 48 grams of lecithin a day while maintaining a low-fat diet. Lecithin is a natural source of the vitamin choline which is found in high amounts in soybeans, eggs, fish, liver and wheat germ.

•• Fish oils lower levels of cholesterol and other blood fats associated with heart disease (<u>The</u>

New England Journal of Medicine 312:19, 1210-16). However, eating cold-water fish like salmon, trout, mackerel and cod will provide plenty of healthful fish oils without having to take the "possibly dangerous" fish oil supplements (International Journal of Epidemiology 6/86).

In fact, fish oil supplements should be avoided. Supplements can cause diarrhea and increase bleeding time, reports The Medical Letter (29:731). Cod liver oil especially should be avoided because it contains cholesterol and can lead to overdoses of vitamins A and D, according to a report from Dr. Nathaniel Shafer of New York Medical College in the Medical Tribune. Other researchers, including Harry S. Glauber of the University of California at San Diego, report that fish oil capsules can actually raise blood sugar levels in diabetics. People with inactive diabetes may discover that the fish oils activate the problem, Glauber says. He recommends that diabetics and people at high risk for developing diabetes should avoid the supplements.

•• Love may be an important ingredient in the battle against cholesterol. According to a study by Fred Cornhill at Ohio State University, cholesterol levels were lower in rabbits who had been petted and cuddled daily than in rabbits who had not received any special attention. The study, reported in Rodale's <u>Natural</u> <u>Healing</u>, noted that in identical circumstances with an identical diet, the animals who received the "tender loving care" had lower cholesterol levels.

•• Here are some easy ways to help reduce the cholesterol in your diet:

> Check food labels very carefully. Products labeled "low-cholesterol" may not conform to the same standards.

> If you are using egg substitutes in trying to reduce your cholesterol intake, be careful. Many commercial egg substitutes are high in sodium or high in fat, even though they may be cholesterol-free. To reduce cholesterol, <u>Cardiac</u> <u>Alert</u> (9:5) recommends using two egg whites instead of one whole egg in cooking and baking.

> Eliminate one pie crust when baking pies. Make your pies "open-faced" rather than covering them with a second crust.

> Don't use lard, shortening, or animal fat drippings for cooking. Make sure the oil you use for cooking is polyunsaturated like corn, safflower, sesame seed, cottonseed, soybean and sunflower oils. Monounsaturated options like olive oil and peanut oil are even better for your health than polyunsaturated oils, according to recent studies.

> In recipes, reduce the amount of added fat

by one-third to one-half. Make up the difference by adding water. For example, if the recipe calls for one cup of oil, just add 2/3 cup of oil and 1/3 cup water. The next time you make the same recipe, try further reducing the amount of oil. Keep cutting back on the fat until you have reached the "lowest possible" fat level for that recipe.

> Reduce the amount of peanut butter in your diet, or eliminate it entirely.

> Buy lean cuts of meat. Always trim any noticeable fat off of meat and poultry before and after you cook it. Remove the skin from chicken, turkey and fish.

> When eating red meat, serve less meat by preparing dishes that use meat plus vegetables, pasta or grains. Then you can use less meat per person while still providing adequate protein, vitamins and minerals. Stir-frying strips of meat with vegetables or cooking them in a wok is a good example.

> For dishes that require hamburger, substitute ground turkey (without the skin) or, if you are a hunter, you may want to substitute ground venison.

> Don't buy meat, fish or poultry that is already breaded. If you want to bread the meat, make your own breading with plain bread crumbs, herbs, skim milk and egg whites. Don't deep-fry

after breading.

> When making soup, chili, or stew, place the broth in the refrigerator overnight. In the morning, remove any fat that has hardened at the top.

> Eliminate bacon bits from your diet. In salads and soups, try homemade croutons or herbs to add that "spicy" taste.

> Eliminate potato chips, french fries and all fried "fast food" from your diet or pull off all the crisp, breaded portions because they become saturated with cooking oil.

> Eliminating salt and butter or oil on popcorn is not always easy because without the liquid, it seems as if no other herbs or spices will stick to the popcorn. Try this delicious alternative. Lightly spray the popcorn with a "non-stick" vegetable spray, then add cinnamon, curry powder, onion powder (not onion salt), chili powder or other herbs for an enjoyable flavor without cholesterol or salt.

> When buying processed foods, watch for "catch words" on the label that indicate high fat or high cholesterol levels: lard, butter, shortening, fat, cream, hydrogenated or hardened oils, palm, palm kernel oil, coconut oil, whole-milk solids, whole-milk fat, egg solids, egg-yolk solids, suet, animal fat, animal byproducts, cocoa butter, milk

chocolate, or imitation milk chocolate. Avoid these products.

Cold Sensitivity

•• Losing heat from your body can be life-threatening. For a skier, a hiker, a skater, a person stuck in a car in a snowstorm or for an elderly person living alone, staying warm is essential.

•• According to the National Institute on Aging, over 2.5 million older Americans are especially vulnerable to cold sensitivity. The U.S. Government reports that people who are at high risk for suffering from hypothermia (low body heat) are:

> the elderly who are frail or sick
> the very old
> people who live alone or in an isolated area
> the poor (who can't afford adequate heat)
> the homeless
> people who do not shiver or feel the cold
> people on prescription drugs that make them insensitive to cold — anti-depressants, blood-pressure reducers, sedatives, tranquilizers and certain heart drugs.
> people who have kidney problems, overactive thyroids or hypoglycemia.

> alcoholics or people who drink a lot of alcohol.

•• People at high risk for hypothermia should take precautions to stay warm when it's cold.

> Wear loose layers of warm clothing when inside or outside. Wearing layers of clothes will make it easier for you to stay comfortable by adding or removing clothing.

> Do not wear tight clothing or tight jewelry because it can constrict the flow of blood in the body.

> If your hands or feet are cold, add more clothes to your whole body. Use the temperature of your extremities as a guide to your whole body's temperature.

> Use an electric blanket or extra blankets when sleeping.

> If cold is a problem while you are sleeping, consider wearing "long johns", comfortable (not tight) socks and a cap to bed.

> People in wheelchairs should consider a "lap blanket" to keep their legs warm.

> After a bath or shower, dry your body and your hair completely.

> Get enough sleep and rest. If you are tired, your sensitivity to the cold is increased.

> Drink plenty of fluids, but avoid alcohol.

> Do not smoke or use any nicotine-containing product because nicotine constricts your arteries.

> Eat a well-balanced diet.

> Exercise and move around as much as possible. Even someone confined to bed or a wheelchair should keep as active as possible.

> When outside, wear a hat and scarf. Up to half of your body heat can be lost through an unprotected head and neck.

> Cover your ears. Use a hat with "ear flaps" or warm ear muffs.

> Keep dry. Remove wet or damp clothing promptly.

> Wear mittens instead of gloves to keep your hands warmer.

> Wear lined boots that cover the calves of the legs. If you don't own boots, wear shoes that are a little large and wear two pairs of socks.

> To avoid inhaling cold air, place a scarf or mask over your nose and mouth. This will help warm the air before it reaches your lungs. The material may get wet and soggy if you are outside for a long time, so have an extra dry scarf available.

> Don't go outside on cold, windy days since the wind-chill factor may be much colder than the temperature alone.

> If you are living alone, arrange to have someone come and visit you everyday. An accident could prevent you from being able to stay warm, and a daily visit would provide an opportunity to reduce the amount of time you would be overexposed to cold.

> Have your home thoroughly insulated including the attic, ceilings, basement and windows. You may also cover your windows or install storm windows (especially on the north side) to reduce drafts in the winter.

> If finances are a problem, consider heating only one or two rooms of your house. But make sure that you will be satisfied to live ONLY in those rooms throughout the winter. Keep the rest of the house warm enough to keep pipes from freezing.

> Low-income families may be able to get special aid from local or state governments in order to keep their homes warm enough throughout the cold months.

> If poor nutrition is a problem, contact a local agency. They may be able to provide a hot meal service that would give shut-ins regular hot, nutritious meals served in their own homes.

•• If a person is at high risk, be sure to watch him carefully for clues to his body temperature.

Stiff muscles, shivering, trembling, a puffy or bloated face, difficult coordination, slow heart rate, slow breathing, low blood pressure, cool or pale skin, a change in personality and confusion can be caused by a drop in body temperature. Many older people have lost their ability to shiver, so don't just rely on shivering as the main sign of hypothermia.

•• If you suspect someone is suffering from overexposure to cold, call an ambulance or a doctor immediately. If a person's temperature drops below 95° F, it is considered to be an emergency. Cover him with blankets, pillows, extra clothes, towels or whatever is available. However, do not move him because he may be very weak. Do not try to "rewarm" him. Don't give him anything to eat or drink. Do not raise the feet because cold blood from the feet will return to the heart and further lower the temperature of the entire body.

Colds

•• There isn't a cure for the common cold, but there are many simple things that you can do to make yourself more comfortable when you have a cold.

•• Zinc gluconate lozenges placed under the

tongue and slowly dissolved in the mouth every two hours while awake have been reported to speed recovery times in people with the common cold, reports <u>Vitamin</u> <u>Side</u> <u>Effects</u> <u>Revealed</u>. However, zinc supplements taken by mouth and swallowed instead of sucked are reported not to have any benefit in curing colds. Be careful! High doses of zinc can produce liver disease, stomach pain and fever, so don't greatly exceed the Recommended Daily Allowance (**RDA**) of 15 mg.

•• Vitamin C is claimed to cure, prevent or reduce the occurrence of the common cold. Most studies show that taking large amounts of vitamin C may reduce the incidence of colds by 20% or 30%. People who take large amounts of vitamin C have fewer cold symptoms than people who don't take large amounts of the vitamin.

Many medical doctors challenge the use of vitamin C in preventing or treating colds. They say that vitamin C either has little or no effect, or that its effect is the same as that of an antihistamine in reducing cold symptoms, but they do not fight the cold virus.

People who use vitamin C to treat colds usually report best results when they quickly increase the amount of vitamin C they are taking as soon as the first symptoms of a cold appear. Many people, like Dr. Linus Pauling, a Nobel prize-winning biochemist, advocate taking as much as 1000 milligrams every hour and up to 20 grams per day to treat a cold or suppress its symptoms. When symptoms disappear with such large doses of vitamin C, the infection may still be present. We don't recommend this regimen because of possible serious side effects, such as ulcers or meningitis. Vitamin C intake should be gradually reduced over the next 10 days to prevent the cold symptoms from returning.

One theory is that vitamin C helps fight colds and other viruses by increasing the activity of the body's immune system. Studies show that vitamin C does improve the ability of the body to produce interferon and to activate white blood cells, both of which help defend the body from invading microorganisms.

•• Vitamin A may help in the treatment of common colds, according to <u>Vitamin Side Effects Revealed</u>. The recommended daily dietary allowance (RDA) of vitamin A is 5000 International Units (I.U.) for adult males and 4000 I.U. for adult females. Vitamin A is naturally found in liver, cod liver oil, eggs, whole-milk products, broccoli, spinach and other green leafy vegetables.

•• Inhaling warm moist air can help soothe the nose and throat. Doctors recommend avoiding public steam baths or saunas when you have a cold, because your respiratory system is weak, and you could pick up a more severe infection. An easy way to do this at home is to boil some water, place it in a large bowl and cover the bowl and your head with a towel. Breathe in the moist air until the water cools. Be sure to lift the towel and breathe cooler air if the heat becomes too intense. Placing some soothing herbs like mint, chamomile or eucalyptus in the water may also be helpful. CAUTION: don't inhale steam from boiling water. It can cause serious burns.

•• Rest if you feel like you need it. A cold takes a lot of energy from the body so you may feel like curling up and sleeping. According to Ladies Home Journal, psychologists believe that allowing your body to rest is the first step to recovering from the cold.

•• Getting your hair wet will not increase your problems with a cold. Wash your hair, bathe or shower if you feel like it. But be smart . . . don't venture into the cold with wet hair!

•• Avoid drastic temperature changes. If you get cold or wet while out-of-doors, do not immediately jump into a hot shower to raise your body temperature.

•• Avoid decongestants and antihistamines except for small children who may develop ear infections after a cold. These over-the-counter drugs can cause high blood pressure or cause the cold to "rebound" and are not recommended by most doctors. If you feel you must take some medication, use a product with a single purpose rather than an "all purpose" cold product.

•• Avoid hot alcoholic drinks. A hot "rum toddy" is a favorite family "cure" for a cold, but doctors warn that it does not have any proven effect. In fact, the hot alcoholic vapors could cause a headache, harm the tender nasal passages or increase chest congestion.

•• Be especially careful when you are under a great deal of stress or deeply depressed. If you are experiencing extreme pressure in your life, be sure to get extra rest and eat a healthful diet to help increase your body's strength. Research has shown that we are most susceptible to colds and infections when we are emotionally stressed.

•• If you are working in a large office or living with someone who has a cold, be sure to wash your hands often during the "cold" season. Cold germs are usually transmitted by the hands: a handshake, telephones, doorknobs, unwrapped candy, pens or pencils, unwashed cups, toothbrushes, pillow cases, and towels. When you have a cold, wash your hands often with soap and water. Do not touch your nose, face or eyes with your hands. After the cold subsides, wash with disinfectant all items that you commonly use and replace your toothbrush.

•• To avoid spreading the infection, cold sufferers should use disposable plates and utensils. Facial tissues should be immediately discarded, preferably flushed down the toilet.

Constipation

•• Natural methods like increasing the amount of fiber in your diet, drinking eight glasses of water each day, getting regular exercise and relaxing during bowel movements are the best ways to treat and prevent constipation.

•• Cut back on the amount of hot and cold tea you drink. According to the British Medical Journal (3/14/81), excessive tea drinking can cause constipation and colon cancer.

•• Avoid commercial laxatives if at all possible. Frequent use of laxatives can actually cause constipation, because laxatives make the body's natural bowel-movement mechanisms

insensitive. Do not use laxatives if:
> you experience nausea or vomiting
> appendicitis is suspected
> you experience abdominal pain
> the intestine could be obstructed or damaged

•• Avoid laxatives containing danthron. Danthron has been proven to cause colon and liver cancer in animals. It was contained in these common laxatives until May 1987: Modane® (Regular, Mild, Liquid and Plus), Doxidan®, Dorbantyl®, Dorbane®, Guarsol®, Danthron tablets, Key Lax® Laxative Tablets, Docusate Calcium® with Danthron, and DC® with Danthron. The Public Citizens Health Letter (3:4), a Ralph Nader newsletter, suggests that you throw away any laxatives you have which contain danthron, or return them to your pharmacist for a refund. Products containing danthron have been banned in Britain and the United States, but some people may still have these products in their medicine cabinets.

Dandruff

•• <u>The</u> <u>Merck</u> <u>Manual</u> recommends washing your hair with a tar shampoo or a shampoo with zinc pyrithione, selenium sulfide, sulfur and salicylic acid. However, other specialists recommend shampooing daily with a <u>mild</u> shampoo. It is important to change your shampoo for two weeks out of every eight weeks. This may help stop the ingredients in one particular kind of shampoo from building up and damaging your hair and scalp.

•• The publishers of <u>Prevention</u> magazine suggest soaking your hair with warm apple-cider vinegar. After you pour it on your hair, wrap your head with a towel and let the vinegar "set" for about an hour.

•• Several <u>Prevention</u> readers claim that vitamin E rubbed into the scalp has helped their dandruff, although medical studies have not proven it.

•• Dandruff is usually worse in the winter since it can be affected by climatic conditions. Wash your winter hats and scarves often so that dandruff doesn't build up on them and continually affect your scalp.

Dental Problems

•• To effectively remove plaque, you must brush your teeth for at least five minutes, according to new research by the University of Iowa. The study reports that a typical American brushes his or her teeth for only about 30 seconds, so much of the plaque that could be removed is left on the teeth. Be careful! Brushing this much daily can cause severe erosion of the tooth enamel, according to other experts.

•• Get plenty of vitamin D which helps in the development of strong teeth and bones. This is especially important in children because their teeth are developing. The best source of vitamin D is sunshine; the sun's action on the skin naturally forms vitamin D. Food sources of vitamin D include fish, fish-liver oils, liver, eggs, and vitamin D-fortified milk.

•• Bleeding and swelling of the gums, gum infections and tooth infections may be caused by a deficiency of vitamin C. A severe vitamin C deficiency, known as scurvy, could cause the complete loss of teeth. Adequate vitamin C promotes healthy gums by preventing tartar from forming, reports <u>Vitamin</u> <u>Side</u> <u>Effects</u> <u>Revealed</u>. Vitamin C is found naturally in rose hips, acerola cherries, green peppers, parsley, broccoli, brussels sprouts, cabbage, potatoes, and citrus fruits.

•• Low levels of calcium in the blood may contribute to tooth decay, according to Vitamin Side Effects Revealed. Dairy products, leafy green vegetables, salmon, and sardines are the best natural sources of calcium.

•• Mouth diseases and bad breath have been linked to a diet deficient in vitamin B6 (pyridoxine), reports J. Dale Hall, D.D.S. Vitamin Side Effects Revealed notes that vitamin B6 supplements have been used to prevent tooth decay. The recommended daily dietary allowance (RDA) for vitamin B6 for an adult is between 1.2 and 2.2 milligrams. Vitamin B6 is naturally found in yeast, liver, whole-grain products, meat, navy beans, fish and nuts.

•• The mineral phosphorus is important in the formation of teeth. Phosphorus is present in high-protein foods like meat, fish, whole-grain products, eggs, dried fruits, corn and soft drinks. However, too much phosphorus may drive the calcium out of the bone tissue, so beware of drinking too many soft drinks or following a high-protein diet over an extended length of time. Phosphorus deficiency is rare because it is abundant in most diets. It usually occurs in people who use aluminum based antacids which bind phosphorus in the intestines and prevent it from being absorbed.

•• Once permanent teeth come in, fluoride taken into the body has little or no effect in preventing decay, reports Frank W. Cawood in Vitamin Side Effects Revealed. Fluoride is often added to public water supplies. Overdoses can cause chalky white areas on the teeth or brown and pitted teeth. Cawood suggests that after a child's permanent teeth come in, families living in areas where the water is fluoridated should switch to bottled water to prevent overdoses of fluoride and its many proven bad side effects.

•• Breastfeeding your baby may reduce the risk of improper jaw alignment and dental problems later in life, according to dentist Michael Elsohn. Babies who are breastfed must thrust the lower jaw forward to grasp the breast, unlike a bottle-fed baby. The thrusting of the lower jaw improves its development because the muscles that support the lower jaw become stimulated. Children who were breastfed experience fewer orthodontic problems, like overbites, explains Dr. Elsohn.

•• Supplements of vitamin B5 (pantothenic acid) may lower the incidence of teeth-grinding during sleep, known as bruxism. Yeast, whole-grain products, liver, salmon, eggs, beans, seeds, peanuts, mushrooms, elderberries and citrus fruits are good sources of vitamin B5.

•• Drink plenty of water. Water helps to rinse mouths and remove the sugary substances that cause cavities. Cut down on soft drinks or other sweet drinks, and drink more water to reduce your risk of dental problems. Rinse your teeth and mouth with water after drinking fruit juices since they contain high amounts of natural sugar.

•• Sealants are now available to help protect your teeth from cavities. These new sealants are especially effective for children. They are applied to the rough inner or center areas of the teeth in the dentist's office. The sealants can last up to seven years. However, good brushing, flossing and eating habits should be observed even with sealants.

•• If you wear properly fitting dentures, you shouldn't need to use an adhesive, reports George Murrell, D.D.S. of the University of California in Los Angeles. One ingredient in commonly used adhesives is Karaya gum, which can dissolve bone tissue and enamel of remaining natural teeth and may cause fungous infections in the mouth, says Murrell. If you like the "added security" of using an adhesive, he suggests using one without Karaya gum. Check the labels.

•• Many denture wearers complain about not

being able to sleep and suffering from headaches or aching jaws in the mornings. According to an article in <u>American Health</u>, some denture wearers remove their dentures to sleep; this leaves the jaw joints without support. Headaches and insomnia should disappear if the person sleeps with his dentures and removes them for a few hours during the day instead.

Depression

•• Depression can be caused by many factors, according to the U.S. Department of Health and Human Services, including:
> genetic predisposition
> biological imbalances
> personality characteristics
> stressful life events
> culture
> age
> sex
> learned behavior
> social and economic class

•• Many people may not know how to express their deeply depressed feelings, so it is often important to know the physical signs which may accompany major depression:

> frequent crying
> anxiety
> nervousness
> drastic weight loss or weight gain
> feelings of guilt
> helplessness
> difficulty with sleeping
> sadness
> loss of energy
> headaches
> irritability
> slowed speech and movement
> restlessness and hyperactivity
> feelings of worthlessness
> loss of affection
> lack of sex drive
> anger
> loss of self-esteem
> constipation

•• Medical treatment with antidepressants for serious depression can be highly successful if the "right" antidepressant is used. In some cases, three or four antidepressants may have to be tried for a few weeks each before the "right" one which reverses that particular type of depression is found.

Antidepressants are non-addictive drugs which can return a depressed person to a normal range of high, low and medium moods. They are <u>not</u> stimulants. With the exception of manic-depressive illness which is best treated with lithium carbonate or other drugs, over 90% of seriously depressed people can be treated successfully if both the patient and doctor are willing to keep on trying until the "right" antidepressant is found.

•• Many people classified as having serious depression may actually be suffering from undiagnosed thyroid problems, according to Dr. Irl Extein of Fair Oaks Hospital in Boca Del Ray, Florida (<u>Journal</u> <u>of</u> <u>the</u> <u>American</u> <u>Medical</u> <u>Association</u> JAMA 249: 12, 1618-1620). Extein and other researchers have found that up to 10% of "untreatable" depressed people actually have hypothyroidism (low thyroid function) which is not detected by the initial thyroid test. Anyone with serious depression should take a detailed series of thyroid tests, recommends Dr. Extein. The thyroid problems can be treated by medication, and most patients find that the depression is significantly relieved as soon as the thyroid problem is under control, he explains.

•• Women may suffer a depressive reaction to taking oral contraceptives, according to the U.S. Department of Health and Human Services.

Researchers are now exploring the effects of oral contraceptives and premenstrual syndrome (PMS) on depression in women.

•• In some studies on specific types of depression, tryptophan, an amino acid naturally contained in soybeans, nuts, tuna and turkey, seems to reduce depression.

•• One type of depression called Seasonal Affective Disorder (SAD) is related to the lack of light during winter, reports the Mayo Clinic Health Letter (5:3). Many people experience elation during the summer months but begin to feel extremely depressed during the fall as winter approaches. Researchers from the Mayo Clinic use light therapy to help patients through the dark winter months. During treatment for SAD, patients use many fluorescent bulbs for their daily activities. The additional light helps improve many cases of depression, say the doctors. But they warn that if the light therapy stops, the patients will relapse.

•• Doctors at Belmont Hospital in Massachusetts and at Harvard Medical School have shown that lecithin helps depression. Lecithin is a natural source of the vitamin choline which is also found in high amounts in soybeans, eggs, fish, liver and wheat germ. However, choline should NOT be given to people who have manic-depressive psychosis, warns <u>Vitamin Side Effects Revealed</u>. Substances which may increase acetylcholine formation, including choline, tend to worsen this type of depression.

•• Low levels of the B vitamin, folic acid, have been linked to depression by A. Missagh Ghadirian of McGill University in Montreal (<u>Psychosomatics</u>, 11/80). Dr. Ghadirian found that depression was alleviated in people by folic acid supplementation if the depression was caused by low folic acid levels. Folic acid is naturally found in yeast, liver, lima beans, whole-grain products, leafy green vegetables, oranges, asparagus, turnips, peanuts, oats, potatoes, and beans.

•• Mild depression may be helped by growing plants, according to the National Horticultural Therapy Association (<u>Health</u> 19:3). Growing plants seems to help increase people's self-confidence levels, increase their awareness of things other than themselves, and provides a peaceful diversion to their everyday activities.

•• When you feel yourself becoming depressed, evaluate your feelings and see if you can understand the reason why you are depressed. Talk to a good friend or write down what you are feeling. Don't expect the friend to solve your problem. A sympathetic "ear" can help you to feel less alone and can help you to sort out your problems.

•• If you really feel as if you need to "get it out", try screaming in your pillow or in a shower.

•• Distract yourself at the first sign of mild depression or a "bad mood." Sometimes people feel as if they "don't deserve" to be happy, and they punish themselves. Try immersing yourself in an activity you enjoy, like reading, cycling, swimming, yardwork, a TV show or a long distance call to a friend.

•• Mild depression can be caused when events don't go as we planned or thought they should. Be flexible. Consider each event as it happens and enjoy it. If it doesn't meet your desired expectations, you must be willing to "make the best" of the situation as it unfolds. Many times depression is caused because we get in "a rut" and expect everything to proceed in exactly the same way.

•• According to the Dr. Javad Kashani in the American Journal of Psychiatry, it is difficult to diagnose depression in children under six years of age. Kashani suggests watching for unexplained medical symptoms like loss of appetite, tiredness, changes in their sleeping habits and sadness. These symptoms may be the child's only way of expressing his or her depression, says the doctor.

Diabetes
Diabetics should not take fish oil supplements to lower their cholesterol levels. Harry S. Glauber of the University of California at San Diego reports that fish oil capsules can actually raise blood sugar levels in diabetics. People with inactive diabetes may discover that the fish oils activate the problem, Glauber says. He recommends that diabetics and people at high risk for developing diabetes should avoid the supplements until further research can be done. If a diabetic needs to lower cholesterol, eating cold-water fish like salmon, trout, mackerel and cod will provide plenty of healthful fish oils without having to take commercial supplements.

Diarrhea
•• Diarrhea in infants should be treated with the BRAT diet, according to the Harvard Medical School Health Letter (12:5). BRAT is an abbreviation for Bananas, Rice, Applesauce and Toast. Bananas are a good source of sodium and

potassium which are lost during bouts with diarrhea. Gelatin products, Gatorade®, clear soups, saltine crackers, Rice Krispies® cereal, and flat ginger ale are also acceptable, say the doctors.

•• If diarrhea is severe and the child's mouth becomes dry and urination almost ceases, you need to replace the baby's lost fluids to prevent dehydration. See your doctor or go to the emergency room of a hospital at once. Dehydration is life threatening, and severe dehydration can be successfully treated with intravenous fluid replacement. Commercial solutions are also available including Lytren®, Infalyte® and Pedialyte®.

•• For diarrhea in adults some pharmacists recommend drinking Gatorade® and avoiding oily foods and milk.

Endometriosis

•• Endometriosis is an unusual thickening of the lining of the uterus that forms outside the uterus, on the ovaries, in the fallopian tubes, in the bowel, or other abnormal location. It most often occurs in women who have not had children or who have delayed childbirth until after the age of 30. Women in these high-risk categories should have a thorough gynecological exam at least once a year. Endometriosis can lead to difficult menstruation, painful intercourse, and, in severe cases, infertility. Up to 15% of woman are estimated to have endometriosis.

•• A recent study by the National Institute of Child Health and Human Development discovered that an unusual menstrual cycle increases a woman's risk of developing endometriosis. If a woman normally has heavy periods up to seven days in length or a cycle less than 27 days long, she is considered to be at high risk for endometriosis.

•• Regular aerobic exercise, a minimum of two hours per week, helps reduce the risk of developing endometriosis, according to the National Institute study. Other factors that have been considered possible risks in developing endometriosis, like using tampons, douching and obesity, were not shown to affect the rate of endometriosis in this study.

•• Once endometriosis occurs, the treatment depends on the age of the woman and whether or not she wants to have more children. If the woman can become pregnant and breastfeed her baby, the menstrual cycle will be interrupted, and the growth of the endometriosis will be inhibited, according to The Merck Manual. However, since pregnancy is often difficult to achieve if endometriosis is present, drugs or surgery may be recommended.

Epilepsy

•• What should you do if you see someone experience an epileptic seizure? Although most epilepsy is well-controlled through medication, here are some important facts that could help if you see someone have a seizure:

> Do not panic.

> Remember that during a seizure the person is temporarily unconscious and cannot be awakened. Do not try to stop the seizure or restrain the movement.

> The person should be made as comfortable as possible and should be protected from hurting himself.

> Loosen any restrictive clothing, especially in the neck area.

> Remove any potentially dangerous objects from the surrounding area.

> Place a pillow, folded coat or other type of cushion under his head.

> Do not allow the person to lie so that vomit would be swallowed or inhaled. If the person is on his back, move him to his side. Make sure that

vomit and fluids are flowing out of the mouth and not being trapped in the throat.

> Do not allow the person to lie face downward on a soft surface. Move him onto his side.

> If the person is sitting in a chair or other precarious position, move him to the floor or onto a bed.

> Do not attempt to open his mouth or to put anything in the mouth.

> If the person turns blue or the seizure lasts for more than just a few minutes, call an ambulance.

Exercise

•• Regular exercise may help prevent premature deaths in middle-aged men, according to a twenty-year study recently published in The Lancet. However, the researchers found that *heavy* physical activity did not prolong the life span. Physical activity tested in the study included farming, lumbering, walking, bicycling, and skiing.

•• Be careful when using ankle weights. According to fitness expert Sheila Cluff, your risk of injury increases if you wear ankle weights of more than two pounds each during high-impact activities like aerobics or running. Heavy weights can also disturb your balance and cause muscle strain rather than just toning. To avoid damage and increase the effectiveness of your workout, Cluff suggests using light weights and doing additional repetitions of each exercise.

Eye Problems

•• Inflammation of the cornea of the eye is often caused by improperly using or cleaning soft contact lenses. According to James McCulley, M.D. of the Department of Ophthalmology at the University of Texas Medical School, many eye problems could be eliminated if people took proper care of their contact lenses (Journal of the American Medical Association JAMA 258: 18). Here are some cautions:

> If you experience changes in vision, discomfort, redness in the eyes or unusual tearing, contact your eye doctor immediately so any possible problems can be treated quickly. Serious eye infections leading to vision loss can be caused by improper cleaning and care of contact lenses.

> Use only the solutions recommended by your eye doctor. Never use distilled water or tap water, or add salt tablets to water to clean lenses.

None of these is sterile, says Dr. McCulley. He suggests using a commercially prepared, saline solution without additional preservatives for cleaning.

> Do not place contact lenses in your mouth because germs from your saliva can be very harmful to your eyes.

> Do not wear soft contacts when swimming.

> Most important, remember to properly clean your contact lenses regularly as recommended by their manufacturer. *Every time* lenses are removed from the eyes, they should be cleaned before they are replaced in the eyes, says The FDA Consumer.

•• Prescription and over-the-counter eye drops can affect your whole body, not just your eyes. If the drops get into the tear ducts, they can enter your bloodstream and affect your whole body. However, if you keep your eyes tightly closed for three minutes after applying eye drops, most of the medicine will be absorbed by the eyes, reports Modern Medicine (53,11: 22). Eye drops can affect more than your eyes so be sure to realize that they contain potent drugs. Do not abuse them, and tell your pharmacist about any other drugs you are taking.

•• People taking birth control pills or

tetracycline, or those who have recently had cataract surgery should be careful about exposing their eyes to ultraviolet rays since they will experience increased sensitivity to the rays.

•• Eye-makeup can contribute to eye infections by allowing bacteria to get into your eyes. Here are some makeup suggestions from the <u>University of California Wellness Letter</u> (3:9):

> Don't buy or use eye makeup that has already been opened. Never use open eye makeup in "testers" at stores on your eyes. They may be contaminated. Test them on the back of your hand.

> Replace your mascara every two or three months. Mascara kept for many months or years is a common source of bacteria and eye infections.

> Never use saliva to wet eye makeup.

> Always wash your hands before applying eye makeup.

> Never use someone else's eye makeup or applicators. Never allow anyone else to use yours.

> Be careful that you don't scratch your eye when applying makeup.

> Clean or replace all applicators at least every three months.

> If you have an eye infection, don't use eye makeup. Consult your doctor.

Falls

•• Falls are the single most common cause of accidental death in people aged 65 and older. Falls lead to hip fractures which can immobilize and lead to other complications, such as lethal blood clots. Many accidental falls by the elderly may be caused by medication, according to an extensive study by a California pharmacist. In a fourteen-month study, Kerry G. Sobel, Pharm. D. of Northwestern Memorial Hospital, found that specific drug classes are associated with falls of elderly patients in nursing homes. People taking drugs in these classes are at an increased risk of suffering a disabling fall:

> thiazide diuretics
> sedatives
> hypnotics (sleeping pills)

•• Another recent study in The New England Journal Of Medicine (316:7,363-9) found several other drugs that caused an increased risk of hip fractures. Drugs which are slowly excreted by the body were discovered to cause the most falls. Because there is difficulty in passing drugs through the bodies of elderly people, "slow moving" drugs become more harmful, says the report. Most of these medications are mood-altering drugs used in the treatment of depression, insomnia, anxiety, or psychosis:

> amitriptyline (Elavil®, Triavil®)
> chlordiazepoxide (Librium®, Librax®)
> chlorpromazine (Thorazine®)
> diazepam (Valium®)
> doxepin (Adapin®, Sinequan®)
> haloperidol (Haldol®)
> imipramine (Tofranil®)
> thioridazine (Mellaril®)

•• To help prevent accidental falls:

> Avoid using "scatter" rugs in the home. If they are used, tape them to the floor. Make sure that the edges of all rugs, carpets and flooring are securely fastened to the floor.

> Use a bench in your bathtub or shower, so you can sit and shower. Install grab bars in your shower or over your tub. Use adhesive rubber strips to prevent slipping because rubber mats can slide.

> Put adhesive rubber strips on stairs.

> Use handrails whenever possible. Have handrails built for all steps and ramps in your home.

> Put wires and cables behind or under furniture where they will be out of the way.

> Make sure the inside and the outside of your

home are well-lit so you can avoid any obstacles.

> Avoid the use of alcohol. It is another drug that can contribute to dangerous falls.

Feminine Hygiene

•• Good feminine hygiene can help prevent urinary tract infections, vaginitis and other vaginal problems. Many infections can occur from poor hygiene practices without sexual contact.

> If you suspect an infection, make an appointment to see your doctor and do not douche before you go. Douching can make it impossible for the doctor to get a culture of the infection.

> Perfumes and ingredients in douches, toilet paper and feminine deodorant sprays can cause an allergic reaction in many people. If you stop using these products, vaginal irritation may clear up without further treatment.

> If you have an infection, don't douche except on your doctor's instructions. Douching changes the acid level in the vagina, and it is not necessary for good feminine hygiene. Douching increases the risk of developing pelvic inflammatory disease. A study in the <u>American Journal of Obstetrics and Gynecology</u> suggests that douching should be completely avoided because it can lead to tubal

(ectopic) pregnancies. Many douches contain chemicals that are dangerous to infants, so women who are pregnant or possibly pregnant should also avoid douching.

> Keep your vaginal and anal areas as clean as possible. Wash them at least once a day with soap and water. Wipe from front to back so that material from your bowels does not contaminate the vagina.

> Anything that is inserted into your vagina, like a contraceptive device, should be cleaned before and after use.

> While you are being treated for an infection, avoid sexual intercourse. If you have recurrent infections, your sexual partner should be examined by a doctor because he may be causing the infections.

> Do not use tampons or a diaphragm if you have an infection. Be sure to always remove your tampons and diaphragms promptly. Keeping them in longer than recommended by the manufacturer can cause an infection.

> Avoid skin-tight pants, synthetic underwear and pantyhose. They may cause the vaginal area to retain heat and create the perfect environment for bacteria to breed. If you have frequent vaginal infections, wear cotton underwear and pantyhose with a cotton crotch to allow heat to escape.

> If your doctor prescribes medication for your infection, use it exactly as directed and continue it for as long as the doctor prescribes. Even if the infection appears to subside, the medication should be continued for the full length of treatment so the infection does not return.

> Have a pelvic exam at least once a year so the doctor can check for cancer of the cervix, vaginal infections or any other irregularities.

Fertility   See: Infertility

Fibrocystic Breast Disease

•• A new drug may be the best treatment for severe fibrocystic breasts, reports U.S. Pharmacist (52:5,111). Danazol (Danocrine®), which is similar to the male hormone testosterone, can provide relief from the severe swelling and pain sometimes caused by fibrocystic breasts, according to the journal. However, danazol has many strong undesired side effects, like lowering the voice and other male patterns, so the drug is recommended only in severe cases.

•• A study in Modern Medicine says that women with fibrocystic breast disease should avoid drugs containing methyl-xanthine or caffeine. Anacin®, Aqua-Ban®, caffeine capsules, Coryban-D®, Dexatrim®, Dietac®, Dristan®, Midol®, NoDoz®, and Triaminicin® contain methyl-xanthine. Caffeine is found in coffee, tea, cola and pepper drinks, chocolate, and some drugs.

•• Since women who have breastfed at least one child have lower incidence of fibrocystic breast disease, breast-feeding may lower the risk of developing this painful problem.

•• Good breast support is essential for women with fibrocystic breast disease, so supportive bras should be worn at all times.

•• Oral contraceptives have been prescribed to help balance the hormones and reduce fibrocystic breast disease in some women. However, oral contraceptives seem to worsen the condition in others.

•• Women with fibrocystic breast disease should have a physical exam by a gynecologist and a mammogram at least twice a year. Some types of fibrocystic tissues are associated with a higher risk of breast cancer.

Food Poisoning

•• Food poisoning is quite rare now, due to

good home refrigeration and strict standards within the food industry. However, contaminated food does not usually taste, smell or look any different from regular food. These tips to avoid any possible problems are from the U.S. Department of Agriculture and The Institute of Human Nutrition at Columbia University.

> Make sure that your refrigerator and freezer meet the standards for good food storage. Your freezer should maintain a temperature of 0 °F (-18° Celsius) or lower while your refrigerator should be a minimum of 40°F (5° Celsius) or colder. Check your storage temperatures with a different thermometer at least once a year to ensure safe standards. Check the gaskets and seals of your refrigerator and freezer to avoid leakage.

> Make sure your kitchen, food storage and food preparation areas are extremely clean. Scrubbing brushes, sponges, dishcloths and kitchen towels should be washed and replaced often.

> Clean the inside of your refrigerator and freezer with one tablespoon of baking soda that has been dissolved in one quart of water. Rinse with plain water. Recommended by the Food and Drug Administration (FDA), this method will help prevent the growth of mold.

> When grocery shopping, avoid changes in

food temperatures as much as possible. Put frozen foods and foods that require cold storage in your cart or basket last. Bring the food home quickly from the grocery store. If you are running several errands, do the errands before you purchase any food. If you live many miles from the grocery store, consider bringing an ice chest and storing your most perishable food on ice while you are driving home.

> Do not re-package meat and poultry unless there is a tear or problem with the store's packaging. The more the meat is handled, the higher the risk of its becoming contaminated. If you don't like the wrapping, add your own layer onto it, rather than removing it and exposing the meat to air. Aluminum foil, freezer paper, plastic wrap or wax paper are acceptable wraps. Date all packages so you can use the oldest food first.

> Do not store leftover food in an opened can. Transfer it to another container because the lead seam in the can may contaminate the food, once the can has been opened.

> Chopped meat, like hamburger, has been handled more than other cuts of meat and is most likely to be contaminated. It can spoil much faster than other meat because of dispersal of contamination within the meat during chopping.

Use it within two days or freeze it. Don't use it if it smells unusual. When camping, cook your chopped meat first, and cook it thoroughly to avoid problems.

> Use two chopping boards — one for meat and one for vegetables — to avoid having juice from raw meat contaminating your other foods.

> If you use a lunch box, remove all contents and wash it thoroughly each night. Bags, garbage and leftover food particles can be a good medium for the growth of bacteria which could affect tomorrow's lunch.

> Clean your can opener frequently and thoroughly. As with the lunch box, leftover food particles on it can breed unwanted bacteria.

> Marinating meat does not prevent bacteria from growing, although lemon juice, vinegar or wine marinades may slow the growth. Always marinate meat and poultry in the refrigerator.

> Only buy dairy products, including milk, cheese, and cream, that have been pasteurized.

> Do not eat bruised or moldy fruit because it may contain toxic substances. Cut away any moldy or bruised sections before eating the rest of the fruit.

> Potatoes, carrots and other root vegetables should be thoroughly cleaned and scrubbed to

remove all the dirt from their surfaces. Many organisms that cause food poisoning are present in soil.

> After boiling eggs, cool them in air, not in cold water. Bacteria from the water can penetrate the shell and harm the eggs.

> Freezing does not purify water. Use only clean water for making ice cubes. When traveling in countries where the water is suspect, request bottled or boiled water.

> When camping, boil or use purification tablets for all drinking, cooking and cleaning water.

> Increase the cooking time when using frozen foods. The U.S. Department of Agriculture generally recommends cooking frozen food one-and-a-half times as long as the cooking time for the fresh food. For example, if the fresh food should be cooked for 10 minutes, the frozen food should be cooked for 15 minutes.

> Cook all foods completely. If cooking is interrupted, bacteria could grow.

> When re-heating, be sure to raise the temperature of the food high enough to kill any bacteria that may have developed. For example, don't just "warm" gravy but bring it to a boil before re-serving.

> Do not eat peanuts that are moldy or shriveled.

> Do not eat raw seafood of any kind.

> Only fish and catch shellfish in safe, clean water. Do not eat fish or seafood that comes from polluted or contaminated waters.

> Do not eat green potatoes. Cut off any green sections.

> When picnicking, choose foods that are LEAST likely to spoil. Foods that are moist and contain protein are the most likely to spoil. Avoid foods like eggs, potato salads, meat, poultry, cream pies, shellfish, milk and milk products, gravies, refried beans, cooked sweet potatoes, squash, rice, corn, mushrooms, cake fillings, eclairs, and custards.

> When packing for a picnic, make sure that any uncooked meat or poultry is in an airtight sealer so that none of its juices could contaminate any other food. Do not eat any food if it has been soaked or contaminated by uncooked poultry juices.

> Watch for expiration dates on the packages of food you store at home. An "expiration" date is the last date the food should be used. A "freshness" date means that the food, usually bakery goods, will be freshest before the date but will still be safe to eat after that date.

> Observe the storage method recommended on the food's packaging. Something in a box or a can may need refrigeration.

> On airplanes, avoid seafood cocktails and any hors d'oeuvres that contain aspic. According to the Centers for Disease Control (CDC) in Atlanta, these foods caused the most cases of food poisoning in airline travel last year. Luxury passengers are at a higher risk, says the CDC, since many of their meals are "gourmet" foods that require more careful attention and storage than the food served to passengers in the coach section.

Foot Problems

•• To prevent foot blisters, apply a cream, like petroleum jelly, to the areas on the feet most susceptible, or take a tip from backpackers, and use a small piece of lamb's wool to help protect your heels and other areas where blisters could form. Be especially careful to use protective measures when wearing new shoes or going hiking.

•• Severe heel pain can be helped by wearing shoes with rubber soles and heels, according to the <u>Mayo</u> <u>Clinic</u> <u>Health</u> <u>Letter</u> (5:5). Also, try adding a piece of styrofoam or a soft sponge to your shoes. Be sure to leave a hole cut out of the sponge for your heel. Massage your feet and stay off of them as much as possible until the pain subsides.

•• A mixture of aspirin, lemon juice and water is the solution for calluses on your feet, according to Dr. Suzanne M. Levine, author of My Feet Are Killing Me. Dr. Levine recommends crushing six aspirin into a powder and mixing them with one tablespoon of lemon juice and one tablespoon of water. Rub the paste onto the problem area on your foot. Then, wrap your foot in a plastic bag and a towel to create a warm, moist atmosphere so the paste can penetrate the hard calluses. After 15 minutes, unwrap your foot and gently use a pumice stone to wipe away the hard, dead skin. You may need to repeat this procedure a few times before all of the hard spots are removed. Also, you may need to change the shoes that caused the calluses.

•• To help relieve sweaty feet, Dr. Levine recommends alternate hot and cold soaks. This helps constrict the blood vessels and reduce perspiration, she explains. After a hot water soak, soak your feet in lemon juice and ice cubes; then massage them with rubbing alcohol to reduce sweating.

Allow your shoes to completely dry before wearing them again. Only wear shoes made of natural materials like leather that "breathe" well.

Sprinkle talcum powder in your shoes to help absorb moisture.

Gas

•• The FDA Consumer (21:3) reports that "swallowing air" is the most common cause of stomach gas. To lessen the amount of air you swallow, follow these suggestions:

> Eat slowly by putting your knife and fork down between bites. This will slow down your eating and reduce the amount of air you swallow with each bite.

> Don't chew gum. Chewing gum increases the amount of air swallowed.

> Have your dentures checked. Dentures that do not fit properly can add to the amount of air you swallow.

•• Avoid foods known to cause gas problems. According to The FDA Consumer, these foods cause the most gas problems: beans, bagels, bran, broccoli, brussels sprouts, cabbage, cauliflower, and onions.

Apples, apricots, breads, bananas, carrots, celery, citrus fruits, eggplant, prune juice, radishes, and raisins can cause moderate amounts of gas, reports the FDA.

•• Avoid soft drinks and beer. These beverages contain carbon dioxide which can cause gas within your body.

•• Avoid milk and dairy products if you have lactose-intolerance. (Lactose is a natural enzyme within the body, necessary for digesting milk).

•• Avoid foods with a high fat content because they can slow down the digestive system and create more of a gas build-up.

•• The FDA has also tested several folk remedies which they discovered to have "no effect" in relieving gas problems. These include the blessed thistle plant, dehydrated garlic, ox bile, and the roots of the golden seal plant.

Gum Disease

•• Gum disease can lead to the loss of your teeth, even if you brush after every meal and see your dentist every six months. Here are some of the warning signs of gum disease, called gingivitis, prepared by the American Dental Association. If you have any of these warning signs, see your dentist:

> Your toothbrush becomes pink or red, or if you notice bleeding of your gums during brushing.

> You seem to be getting "long in the tooth"

because your gums are receding.

> Your gums are sore, swollen, or red.

> You have any pockets of pus developing on your gums.

> You have abnormally bad breath or a unusual taste in your mouth.

> Your teeth seem to be fitting together differently.

> Your dentures or partials fit differently than normal.

> You have new gaps between your teeth.

> You have any loose teeth.

•• Applying the folate form of the B vitamin, folic acid, directly to your gums may help relieve the swelling and pain of gum disease, according to a study by the New Jersey Medical School published in <u>General</u> <u>Dentistry</u> (July 86). Since a deficiency of folate or folic acid is known to cause tender gums, the researchers tested taking oral folate supplements or applying a folate solution directly to the gums. The supplements made only a minor difference, but the direct application reduced the gum pain substantially. Folate is found naturally in yeast, liver, lima beans, whole-grain products, leafy green vegetables, asparagus, beans, turnips, peanuts, oats, potatoes and oranges. To apply folate directly to the gums, a special folate solution would have to be purchased or made.

Hair Care

•• Chlorine in swimming pools can damage normal hair as well as hair that has been permed or colored. According to <u>American Health</u> (6:4), you should rinse your hair immediately after exposure to chlorine. Hair that hasn't been permed or colored should be rinsed with water, shampooed and conditioned. People with permed hair should wear a bathing cap when swimming in chlorinated water. People with tinted hair should rinse it with bottled water or club soda immediately after exposure to chlorine. If tinted hair turns green, treat it with a hot-oil conditioner.

•• All types of hair should be covered to prevent exposure to the sun. The sun dries out hair and causes it to become damaged and brittle. Wear a scarf or hat to protect it. Straw hats allow sunlight to filter through, so they will not fully protect your hair.

Hair Loss In Women

In many cases, hair loss in women is linked to another problem in their overall health. Philip

Kingsley, a specialist in hair problems, says that hair loss in women can often be reversed if the source of the problem can be discovered and treated.

> Gradual hair loss can be caused by anemia due to a lack of iron in the blood. Anemia is quite common in women and can be easily treated by a diet high in iron or by taking appropriate iron supplements, says Kingsley. Iron is naturally found in whole-grain products, liver, organ meats, red meat, eggs, lima beans, prunes, spinach, raw broccoli, peas, fish and raisins.

> A poor diet can cause hair loss. Women who have suffered from anorexia or bulimia or who have eaten a nutritionally deficient diet over a long period of time can suffer hair loss. Resuming a proper diet will help restore normal hair growth.

> Traction hair loss is very common, especially in black women and men, Kingsley reports. It is caused by pulling the hair very tightly over many years. Corn rows, pig tails, ponytails or any other severe hair style can cause the hair line to recede. Reducing the stress on the hair should help.

> Ovarian cysts have been linked to hair loss, says Kingsley. Sometimes hair loss, combined with oily skin and hair growth on other parts of the

body, helps to identify an ovarian problem. However, once the cysts have been properly treated, hair growth resumes as usual.

> Constant twisting or pulling on the hair due to psychological problems or habit can also lead to hair loss. Some young women or older women going through menopause consiously or unconsiously pull their hair to get attention. Psychotherapy to help the mental problems is the only way to break the cycle and let the hair relax, reports Kingsley.

> Bald patches are experienced by about two percent of the general population. In about 98% of these cases, the hair growth will resume and the bald spots will disappear.

> Stress can affect hair growth, so worrying about hair loss can just add to the problem. Kingsley suggests that most hair loss in women is just temporary. After checking with your doctor, starting on a proper diet, and stopping any damaging hair treatments, you should be able to relax and assume the hair loss is temporary.

Headaches

•• A report in a British journal claims that breathing into a paper bag, considered a cure for hiccups, may also help shorten certain migraine headaches. The paper bag must cover both the mouth and the nose. Exhale into the bag, then breathe from the bag. Repeat several times. The researchers are not sure why it works, although the exhaled air is usually high in carbon dioxide content.

•• Breathing pure oxygen helps reduce the frequency of cluster headaches, according to the <u>Journal</u> <u>of</u> <u>the</u> <u>American</u> <u>Medical</u> <u>Association</u> (JAMA 256:3349). People who suffer from severe cluster headaches may want to keep a tank of oxygen available at home and at work. A traditional oxygen tent is not necessary. The researchers report that just breathing the oxygen through a mask is sufficient.

•• Headaches are a common side effect of many prescription and over-the-counter drugs including:

> Aldactazide® (spironolactone and
                hydrochlorothiazide)
> Aldomet® (methyldopa)
> Demi-Regroton® (reserpine)
> Deprol® (meprobamate)
> Diupres® (reserpine)
> estrogen
> Equanil® (meprobamate)

> HydroDIURIL® (hydrochlorothiazide)
> Hydropres® (reserpine)
> Indocin® (indomethacin)
> Miltown® (meprobamate)
> oral contraceptives
> Regroton® (reserpine)
> Salutensin® (reserpine)
> Ser-Ap-Es® (reserpine)
> Valium®

•• If you suffer from headaches only on weekends, evaluate the amount of coffee you drink during the week. Since the caffeine in coffee constricts the blood vessels, on a morning that you don't drink coffee, a headache may result from the dilated blood vessels. Either reduce the amount of coffee you drink during the week or get up earlier on the weekends and drink your usual amount of coffee.

•• Many headaches due to a hangover can be prevented by eating fatty foods before drinking, limiting your alcohol, and by drinking only light-colored alcohol. Once a hangover headache appears, try eating food high in fructose, like tomato juice or honey, to help neutralize the alcohol. Get extra sleep, drink coffee and rest to help ease the headache.

•• Be wary of sudden or severe headaches.

Research at the University of California at San Francisco has shown that a sudden, severe headache may be the only warning sign of a brain aneurysm, when a blood vessel in the brain develops a weak spot that could explode and cause death. If you experience a "thunderclap" headache or a headache that is sudden and severe for you, call your doctor immediately.

Hearing Problems

•• Adequate beta-carotene, vitamin A and zinc may be important for your hearing. Low blood levels of beta-carotene, vitamin A and zinc have been linked to hearing loss in studies by Erwin Lohle of the University of Freiburg in Germany.

•• A low-cholesterol diet that is good for your heart and arteries may also prevent hearing loss, according to a study in Finland recently published in The Laryngoscope. The researchers discovered that cholesterol limits the amount of blood that flows through the small arteries in the ear, and hearing loss develops. In a study of 4,000 people, hearing improved on a low-fat diet but worsened when fatty foods were given. See our section on **Cholesterol Reduction** for information on how to lower your cholesterol intake.

•• Magnesium deficiency has also been linked to poor hearing, according to research in the Journal of the Acoustical Society of America. Loud noises actually lower the amount of magnesium in the ear. This causes the blood vessels there to constrict which leads to increased hearing loss.

•• Ringing in the ears, known as tinnitus, may be helped by proper nutrition, says Paul Yanick, executive director of the Hearing and Tinnitus Help Association. Yanick believes that proper nutrition creates a chemical balance which helps to stabilize ear sounds.

Heart Problems

•• Up to 60% of Americans are at risk of developing coronary heart disease because they are physically inactive, according to the Morbidity and Mortality Weekly Report by the Centers for Disease Control. Although researchers are not sure exactly how much exercise is needed, they believe that inactivity is a risk as great as high levels of cholesterol, high blood pressure or smoking.

•• A recent study at the University of Pittsburgh found that the true relationship between exercise and prevention of heart disease was the regularity of exercise. They discovered that mailmen who walked an average of five miles a day had higher blood levels of HDL's (the good, protective type of cholesterol). Since the walks were continuously interrupted, the exercise could not be classed as aerobic. The researchers felt that the key was exercising every day rather than being inactive.

•• Avoid coffee, or limit yourself to two cups a day, if you have heart problems. Excessive coffee drinking is known to cause an increased risk of coronary artery disease, angina and sudden heart attack (New England Journal of Medicine 315:16, 977-82). But according to Cardiac Alert (8:5), coffee can also overstimulate the heart and decrease the effectiveness of certain angina and blood-pressure medications. The caffeine in coffee causes an increase in the heart rate which can be very dangerous to someone with heart problems. Cardiac Alert recommends that all coffee, with or without caffeine, should be avoided by people with heart or artery problems.

•• Quit smoking anything! Switching from cigarettes to cigars does not help reduce your risk of having a heart attack, reports the British Medical Journal (6/15/87). Smoking five cigars a day still increases your risk of heart attack by 4.5

times the risk of a nonsmoker, according to the research.

•• A "strong belief in a supreme being" may lower your risk of heart disease, according to a study published in the International Journal of Cardiology (1/86). The study of over 500 men and women found that devout Jews had lower heart-attack rates than non-practicing Jews. In the researchers' own words, "the strong belief in a supreme being and the role of prayer may in themselves be protective."

•• People at high risk for heart problems do just as well taking medicine as they would with major surgery, reveals a new study by Dr. Robert Luchi at the Veterans Administration Medical Center in Houston. People with unstable angina, who are considered at high risk for heart disease, were treated with either heart bypass surgery or with medicine. Dr. Luchi found that both groups had a similar rate of heart attacks. Since drug treatment is less traumatic and less expensive than surgery, the report suggests that drug therapy should be the treatment of choice. However, the researchers warned that the hearts of the people who took medicine were less efficient pumps than those of the people who had received heart surgery. (The New England Journal of Medicine 316: 16, 977-

84).

•• Men with heart disease have high blood levels of Immunoglobulin E (IgE), a substance related to allergies, reports Dr. Michael Criqui in the <u>American Journal of Medicine</u> (6/1/87). The blood levels of IgE were up to 119% higher in men who had coronary heart disease than in men without heart problems. There was no difference in the IgE levels in women with or without heart disease. Whether men with allergies are at higher risk of developing heart disease is not known. The study did not show how heart disease and high IgE levels are related, but Dr. Criqui is planning to do further research on the subject.

•• Some scientific studies have indicated a high incidence of a creased earlobe associated with the development of heart disease. However, a recent study in the <u>Archives of Internal Medicine</u> (147:65-66) reports that the incidence of earlobe crease and the incidence of heart disease both increase with age. The study questioned the relationship between the two conditions. If you have or develop creased earlobes, do not feel that they necessarily mean that you have heart disease.

•• Women who have their ovaries removed should have estrogen-replacement therapy to lower their risk of heart disease, reports <u>The New</u>

England Journal of Medicine (316: 1105-10). Women who had their ovaries removed and did NOT take estrogen had twice the risk of developing heart disease, according to the study conducted at Harvard Medical School.

•• A new blood test could help identify people at high risk of developing heart disease, reports American Health (6:4). The blood test is under consideration for approval by the Food and Drug Administration (FDA). The test is manufactured and developed by California Biotechnology. It can identify certain factors that are known to affect heart disease including:

> cholesterol receptors that control the levels of low and high lipoprotein levels (LDL's and HDL's)

> molecules, called apolipoproteins, that carry blood cholesterol

> certain hormones related to blood pressure

> insulin production levels

•• Portable defibrillators, like the machines used in hospital emergency rooms to "shock" the heart into restarting, could save thousands of lives. The defibrillator delievers a specified amount of electric current to a heart with an irregular heartbeat.

Thousands of Americans suffer from heart

attacks every year and are considered at high risk for having another heart attack. Dr. Richard O. Cummins, a researcher at the University of Washington, explains that the defibrillators could be used by family members, office workers, airline attendants, and rural emergency services. Dr. Cummins explained that CPR (cardiopulmonary resuscitation) helps keep a person alive until the heart can be restarted, but many times the person dies before they can receive medical assistance. Spouses and co-workers of people at high risk for heart attacks can receive just four hours of training and be able to use a portable defibrillator. Portable defibrillators are now approved and available in the U.S. but must be prescribed by a doctor.

•• Your working conditions may be increasing the severity of your heart problems, Dr. Jorge C. Rios warns in Cardiac Alert (8:5). Breathing polluted air in your workplace, working in extremely hot temperatures, working under stress, and working with high noise levels can contribute to heart problems and angina, says Dr. Rios.

•• Sudden bursts of energy are very hard on the heart and arteries and should be avoided. Shoveling snow should be avoided by people with heart problems. Using a snow blower or hiring someone else to shovel on your property is best.

However, if you feel you must shovel the snow by hand, please take these precautions as recommended by <u>Cardiac</u> <u>Alert</u> (8:2):

> Lift with your thighs and legs rather than just using your arms.

> Lift only small loads of snow.

> Pacing yourself is important. Start off slowly to avoid over-exerting your heart to a "sudden burst of energy."

> Don't attempt to do a large job all at one time. Take breaks and relax. Don't push yourself.

> Wear loose layers of warm clothing. Layers will make it easier for you to add or remove clothing. Keep dry, and remove layers of wet clothing. Avoid becoming overheated because that places additional strain on your heart.

> Do not wear tight clothing or tight jewelry because it can constrict the flow of blood in the body.

> Always wear a hat and scarf. You can lose up to half of your body heat through your head and neck if you don't dress properly.

> Cover your ears. Use a hat with "ear flaps" or warm ear muffs.

> Wear mittens instead of gloves to keep your hands warmer.

> Wear lined boots that cover the calves of your legs. If you don't own boots, wear shoes that

are a little large with two pairs of long socks.

> To avoid inhaling cold air, place a scarf or mask over your nose and mouth and breathe through it. This will help warm the air before it enters your lungs. However, the material will get wet and soggy if you are outside for a long time. Have an extra dry scarf available to change when needed.

> Don't shovel on windy days since the wind-chill (the temperature plus the wind-chill factor) may be much colder than the temperature alone.

Also see: **Cholesterol Reduction**.

Heat Stress

•• The U.S. Government reports that certain people are at a high risk of suffering from heat stress including those who:

> are over 65 years of age
> have diabetes
> have cystic fibrosis
> are overweight
> have heart problems
> have had a stroke
> have circulation problems
> are taking diuretic drugs
> are taking drugs for Parkinson's disease

•• Heat stroke is a result of the body's inability to regulate the body's heat. Less serious heat exhaustion is caused by an excessive loss of body fluids, according to The Merck Manual.

If heat stroke is suspected (hard rapid pulse, very high body temperature, hot dry skin), the person should be immersed in cold water or ice and emergency medical services should be contacted immediately. Do not allow the person's temperature to drop below normal.

If heat exhaustion is suspected (pale clammy skin, weak slow pulse, faintness and low blood pressure) the lost fluids need to be replaced, and the person should rest flat or with head between knees. Drink lots of water or mineral replacement beverages like Gatorade®, eat some highly salted food (like nuts or potato chips) and contact the doctor.

•• Heat exhaustion and heat stroke may be prevented by proper care and planning. Take the following precautions during hot weather, particularly if you are in any of the high-risk categories:

> Wear loose, comfortable clothing that covers your shoulders. Lightweight, light-colored clothing is best. Make sure that everything is loose, including your underwear. Loose clothing will help

the air circulate and will keep you cooler.

> Wear a hat when in the sun or carry an umbrella. However, remember to take the hat off when you are in the shade because heat will be able to escape through your head. If you leave your hat on, you may risk heat build-up.

> Stay in air-conditioned places during the heat of the day. If you cannot afford an air-conditioner, visit a library, shopping mall, community center, movie theater, church, museum or other place that is air-conditioned.

> Use fans to help circulate air during the day and to draw in cooler air in the evenings.

> Avoid extended outdoor activities, especially in the heat of the day. Plan outdoor events for the early morning or evening. Avoid long periods of swimming, snorkeling, boating, surfing, water skiing and other outdoor water sports. Although the water will help you feel comfortable, you may be receiving too much exposure to the sun and could still suffer from heat exhaustion.

> If you are exercising during hot weather, as part of your regular fitness program, you may want to drink Gatorade® or another product that helps replace salts, minerals and electrolytes.

> Rest or do "quiet" activities as much as

possible. Exercise or physical activity in hot weather will put additional strain on your heart.

> Drink at least eight glasses of water a day whether or not you are thirsty. Water is better than any other drink to help your body maintain a healthy temperature. Do not drink alcohol because it causes a quick loss of body liquids. If you have a medical problem that is affected by drinking a large quanity of fluids, ask your doctor how much liquid you should be drinking every day.

> Do not eat hot foods or heavy meals. Eat plenty of fresh fruit and vegetables. As well as providing good nutrition and fiber, fresh fruit will add to the water your body receives.

> Consider soaking in a tub of cool water every evening. Avoid hot baths or showers because they increase your body temperature.

> Avoid suntanning. As well as unnecessarily raising your body temperature, exposure to the sun is known to cause skin cancer.

> Your body needs time to adjust to extreme temperatures. If summer comes quickly and the temperature is unseasonally hot, you need to be more careful than later in the summer. If you travel to a tropical climate from a cooler climate, allow your body time to adjust.

Hoarseness

•• Losing your voice can be a frustrating experience, but it can also be a warning sign of medical problems, says the American Academy of Otolaryngology (head and neck specialists). Hoarseness can be related to a simple problem like a cold or abuse of your vocal cords, but it can also be a warning sign of cancer of the larynx (voice box). If you suffer from persistent hoarseness, check with your doctor.

•• To prevent hoarseness or abuse of your vocal cords, Jan Brenner of Executive Voice Control suggests:

> Teach yourself to speak and shout from the stomach, using your diaphragm, rather than from your throat.

> Keep your chin down when shouting. Don't stretch the neck.

> When attending sporting events, clap or whistle rather than shouting. Use a megaphone if you want to make loud vocal sounds.

> Avoid situations where loud music or noise forces you to shout.

> Don't smoke. Don't expose yourself to smoke-filled places.

> Reduce the amount of dairy products you eat

because they can cause thick mucus in the nose and throat.

> Reduce the amount of caffeine you consume.

> Avoid alcohol.

> Suck on a lemon or lemon candy when you are in a situation where you could abuse your vocal cords, like at an exciting football game.

> Drink hot tea with lemon to help soothe your throat.

> Keep your throat moist by using a humidifier or vaporizer in your home or boil water to increase humidity in the winter. Also see our report on **Colds** in this book.

Hyperactivity

•• Hyperactivity in children has often been blamed on high consumption of sugar. However, recent studies have shown that sugar, like other carbohydrates, actually causes people to become sleepy, not overactive.

•• Other researchers suggest that additives from highly processed foods may be causing an "allergic reaction" in hyperactive children. They suggest putting the child on a natural diet of unprocessed foods that are prepared simply.

Although many parents report great success with the natural diet, some doctors believe that the extra attention of getting the special food also helps the child. A massive government study failed to show any strong link between food additives and hyperactivity in children.

The home atmosphere does not necessarily "create" a hyperactive child, but good parenting skills may help a child to overcome hyperactivity.

Indigestion

•• Avoid comfrey-pepsin capsules available for "indigestion" in health food stores. According to <u>The New England Journal of Medicine</u> (315:17,1095) comfrey roots contain a substance known as pyrolizidine which can lead to liver problems and cancer. The journal warns that taking comfrey-pepsin capsules over a period of several months could be very dangerous.

•• Do not take antacids if you are taking prescription medication or aspirin, according to <u>The Medical Letter Handbook of Drug Interactions</u>. Antacids react with many other types of medication, so discuss it with your pharmacist or doctor before you take antacids with:

> benzodiazepines, like clorazepate

> cimetidine (Tagamet®)
> corticosteroids
> digoxin
> fluoride
> indomethacin (Indocin®)
> isoniazid
> pseudoephedrine
> ranitidine (Zantac®)
> salicylates, like aspirin
> tetracyclines, oral
> thiazide diuretics, like Diuril® and Hygroton®

•• Many cases of heartburn and indigestion are caused by yeast but remain undiagnosed, says Dr. Sherry A. Rogers of Syracuse, New York. She says that a yeast-free, sugar-free diet can help relieve the digestive problems caused by yeast.

Infertility

•• Couples who smoke have decreased chances of conceiving and carrying a child to a full-term pregnancy, according to Dr. Michael Rosenberg. Men who smoke have a lower sperm count, less sperm mobility, and more abnormal sperm than non-smoking males, Rosenberg discovered. In women who smoke, spontaneous abortions (miscarriages) occur in 27 out of every 100 conceptions.

•• According to the <u>FDA</u> <u>Consumer</u> (17:5), certain women can solve their fertility problems by douching with water and baking soda just prior to intercourse. Some women have "overly acidic cervical secretions" which can kill the sperm, reports the FDA (Food and Drug Administration). By douching with water and baking soda, the acidic secretions can be neutralized and some sperm can live long enough to fertilize the egg.

Acidic secretions can be detected during a post-coital exam by a gynecologist. Within a few hours after sexual intercourse, the gynecologist can take a scraping from the woman's cervix to see if enough sperm are reaching the cervix.

Kidney Problems

•• Kidney dialysis patients should take a half an aspirin a day to reduce the risk of dangerous blood clots, according to a study at Washington University in St. Louis. The researchers said that the risk of developing a blood clot was reduced by 50 percent when just half an aspirin was taken daily. If you're on dialysis, this should be discussed with your doctor to see if aspirin treatment would be appropriate for you.

Lead Poisoning

•• Lead poisoning can damage the brain, bones, kidneys, liver, central nervous system and immune system and even cause slow-learning in children. A recent study in The New England Journal of Medicine (316: 4/87) found that children who were exposed to high lead levels before birth were physically and mentally impaired during their first two years of life.

•• If lead poisoning is suspected, a doctor or hospital should be contacted immediately. According to The Merck Manual, these are some of the initial symptoms of lead poisoning: headaches, irritability, changes in personality, loss of appetite, constipation, abdominal pain, upset stomach, vomiting, and seizures.

•• Many cases of lead poisoning are caused by frequent use of an everyday item, like a coffee mug, that is cracked or improperly glazed and allows lead to leach into your beverage, especially if you drink acidic beverages. Learn what causes lead poisoning and how to prevent it:

> Do not use glazed pottery for cooking or serving food, unless you know that the glaze does

not contain lead.

> Do not store highly acidic foods or beverages in ceramic ware. The acid in the food or drink reacts with the glaze and increases the lead content of the food. The Merck Manual especially warns about the storage of wine, cider, fruits, fruit juices, tomatoes, tomato juice, and cola drinks because they are highly acidic.

> Do not use pottery or leaded glass from local craftspeople to serve or store food. Beware of imported pottery. The Food and Drug Administration (FDA) has regulated the lead content in serving ware, pewter, enamelware and pottery since the early 1970's. However, many ceramic products that are imported into the U.S., souvenir plates, or products made by local craftspeople may not meet the safety standards. Plates with high lead content can be used "for decorative purposes only" but should not come in contact with food.

> Be careful with antiques like toys, baby cribs, and serving dishes. Old baby cribs may have been painted with lead paint. Have them stripped and repainted if you want to use them — but only after making sure the width between the crib rails is narrow enough to meet current safety standards to prevent accidental choking. Do not allow your

child to play with an old toy that may have been painted with lead paint. Antiques that have questionable lead content levels could be used as decorations on display, but not around children who could put them into their mouths.

> The lead content in paint is now carefully regulated, but paint on the walls, moulding and bannisters of old homes, could contain high levels of lead. Children and pregnant women should avoid remodeling of older homes where high levels of lead may be found. Do not burn painted boards in an indoor fireplace or woodstove, because the lead from the paint would be dispersed into the air.

> Be especially careful with children. Young children often put anything in their mouths, including old paint chips and dirt containing lead. This year it is estimated that 2,000 children just in the state of Massachusetts will suffer from lead poisoning.

> Do not allow your child to swallow any item containing lead, like a fishing sinker, gun shot, or curtain weight. If you know a child has swallowed an item containing lead, contact your doctor immediately.

> If you live in an older home and have soft water, have the lead level of your drinking water tested by the local EPA (Environmental Protection

Agency). Soft water is slightly acidic and can leach lead from old pipes or fittings in and connected to your home. Evan T. Smith, a mechanical engineer from Idaho, suggests running tap water for a few minutes before using it because stagnant water has the highest lead content. By just flushing the pipes with fresh water, you will be able to use water with a lower lead content.

> Don't use hot tap water for preparing baby formulas, drinking or cooking, the Wellness Letter from the University of California at Berkeley recommends. Lead is leached into hot water faster than cold water, the newsletter reports.

> People who repair car radiators have been lead-poisoned due to poor ventilation and a lack of safety procedures, reports the New England Journal of Medicine (317: 214-8). The doctors warn that anyone working in auto repairs should properly ventilate the work area and take breaks outdoors at least once each hour.

> People who manufacture batteries, remodel old homes, or work in smelting are at increased risk of lead poisoning. Be sure to clean these work clothes thoroughly and separately from other clothes. Shower, scrub and change into clean clothes as soon as your work day is over.

> Do not drink homemade wine or whiskey.

Homemade liquor often has a high lead content because facilities and ingredients are not inspected and may not follow lead content standards.

Leg Pain

•• Leg cramps during the night may be alleviated by untucking the covers at the foot of the bed or by placing a small board at the foot of the bed. The board can be used to lift the covers off of the feet and remove that pressure on the toes, when sleeping on your back. It is also useful if the feet are gently rested against the board.

•• If you sleep on your stomach, try letting your feet hang over the bottom edge of the mattress. Your leg muscles will be stretched and relaxed which should reduce the incidence of nightly cramps.

•• A certain type of leg pain, known as intermittent claudication, can be caused when the arteries in the legs become clogged with fatty deposits. This is a serious condition. If the arteries in the legs are becoming restricted, the arteries leading to the heart may also be closing. Your doctor should be contacted for treatment. To help relieve this pain:

> Stop smoking.

> Lose weight.

> Begin a regular exercise program approved by your doctor.

> Rest your legs regularly.

> Eat a low-fat, low-cholesterol diet.

•• Leg pains can be especially dangerous in diabetics. A complete loss of the flow of blood could lead to amputation, so diabetics should SEE THEIR DOCTORS immediately if serious leg pain develops.

Memory Loss

•• Dr. Alexander Reeves, a Dartmouth University researcher, says that staying mentally active is the key to keeping a good memory. Reading, social events, and challenging your mental skills will help keep your memory in good working order. A proper diet, regular exercise, and regular checkups with your physician will help keep you in overall good health, including mental alertness.

•• Remaining sexually active, even in old age, may be a key to a better memory, according to a study by Lar Nilsson, M.D. of Göteborg, Sweden. "A drop in memory capacity and intellectual ability" occurs when you become sexually inactive, reports Dr. Nilsson. A sexually active life is essential for a good memory and a healthy life, he concluded. However, cause and effect may not be proven by his study. Many celibate, religious people retain good intellects in advanced age.

Osteoporosis

•• Salmon calcitonin may be the best new therapy to prevent the loss of bone known as osteoporosis. Calcitonin is a natural hormone that helps bones develop in humans and other animals. Bone mineral content increased by 13% in women who were given calcitonin and calcium compared to women who received calcium and a placebo. Calcitonin could replace estrogen as the "treatment of choice" for osteoporosis because of its effectiveness and because calcitonin has fewer negative side effects than estrogen therapy, according to researcher Dr. Charles Chesnut from the University of Washington in Seattle.

•• Caffeinated-coffee drinkers lose twice as much calcium as people who drink decaffeinated coffee, reports Dr. Linda K. Massey at Washington State University. Caffeine causes calcium to be excreted in urine rather than be absorbed by the body. Dr. Massey suggests that since many coffee drinkers are not getting enough calcium to begin with, drinking coffee containing caffeine is making their problem worse. Massey suggests that if you must drink coffee, drink decaffeinated coffee with lots of milk. The additional milk will help replace some of the calcium that the body needs (<u>Prevention</u> 39:5).

•• Exercise can help strengthen the bones of older women, the Jewish Hospital in St. Louis reports. Until now, many experts believed that weight-bearing exercise could help prevent osteoporosis only before menopause. The new research shows that even women with osteoporosis who are past menopause can benefit from weight-bearing exercise combined with an adequate intake of calcium. Weight-bearing exercise includes activities like aerobics, dancing, walking, jogging, rowing, hiking, rope jumping, tennis or bicycling, where the bones have to support body weight.

Ovarian Cysts

Using oral contraceptives reduces the risk that a woman will develop ovarian cysts, the <u>British Medical Journal</u> reports. Women who use birth-control pills are less likely to develop ovarian cysts or get cancer of the ovary, according to the study.

Pain

•• Eating spicy foods may help to relieve pain. Foods seasoned with capsaicin, the substance that makes chili peppers hot, actually increase the amount of natural painkillers secreted by our bodies. Capsaicin triggers the secretion of endorphins, the body's own painkillers. University of Pennsylvania researcher Paul Rozin, Ph.D., is hoping to discover how capsaicin can be used to relieve pain.

•• For pain caused by overusing muscles or joints, the American College of Sports Medicine (American Health 6:4) recommends:

> Rest the joint or muscle for at least 24 hours.

> Apply ice in a plastic bag or towel for about 30 minutes.

> After the ice treatment, the joint or muscle should be wrapped and elevated for 30 minutes. Then unwrap the problem area, but keep it elevated as much as possible.

> Over-the-counter pain relievers can be taken. Remember that acetaminophen is a good pain-reliever, but does not reduce inflammation like aspirin or ibuprofen products.

Pregnancy

•• Do not drink alcohol while you are pregnant. Just one glass of wine, one can of beer or two cocktails a week could increase by 30% the chances of harming the unborn baby or having a spontaneous abortion (miscarriage). Children born to mothers who drink heavily can be born with fetal alcohol syndrome.

•• Exercise during pregnancy is important, but it should be done with caution to protect both the mother and the baby. The hormonal changes of pregnancy affect the stretchiness of the mother's ligaments and can also cause an elevated heart rate. To avoid problems, the American College of Obstetricians and Gynecologists recommends:

> Wear a very supportive bra.

> Wear supportive, non-slip shoes. The hormonal changes in the body will cause your ligaments to be more relaxed, and you will be more likely to suffer a sprain or other injury.

> Drink plenty of fluids to avoid overheating and dehydration. Drink at least one extra glass of water for every hour you exercise.

> Do not allow your body temperature to rise above 102°F. Do not exercise outdoors in

extremely hot or humid weather.

> Do not increase your heart rate past 140 beats per minute.

> Warm up thoroughly before exercising. Work up to aerobic activity very slowly.

> Twisting, bouncing, and jarring activities should be avoided. Reduce or eliminate bouncing in your aerobic workout. Change to low-impact aerobics throughout your pregnancy, especially during your final trimester.

> Do not do any exercise that causes you to feel uncomfortable. Avoid exercises that involve your abdomen.

> After your fourth month, do not do any exercises lying flat on your back because the blood supply to the baby may become blocked. Lie on your side when needed.

> Avoid holding your breath while exercising.

> If you become dizzy, lose your breath or get tired, stop exercising and rest.

> Do not participate in contact sports.

> Do not play tennis or any other sport that requires sudden stops and starts.

•• Wear your seat belt while you are pregnant. Many women stop wearing their seat belts during their pregnancy because they feel it may hurt their babies. However, more unborn babies die in car accidents because their mothers are NOT wearing their seat belts, reports the Journal of Reproductive Medicine (1/86).

•• Half an aspirin a day can reduce the rate of preeclampsia. Toxemia of pregnancy, known as eclampsia or preeclampsia in its early stages, is a life-threatening condition which occurs in late pregnancy. Dr. Henk Wallenberg of Erasmus University Medical School in The Netherlands discovered that a low daily dose of aspirin will "significantly reduce" the occurrence of preeclampsia in high-risk women. Check with your own doctor about this new research before taking aspirin.

•• Women actively trying to conceive should be taking special care of their health, according to doctors at the University of North Carolina medical school (American Health 6:5).

> Have a check-up so your doctor can identify any physical problems that could interfere with a healthy pregnancy, like urinary tract infections, sexually transmitted diseases, and ovarian cysts. Any diseases that occur in your family history and could be genetically transferred to the child should be reviewed.

> Do not get overheated. Vigorous exercise, hot baths, saunas or hot tubs can cause a dramatic

increase in your body temperature which can harm an unborn child. Since the fetus is particularly sensitive to heat in the first few weeks of development, you should especially avoid becoming overheated while you are trying to conceive and during the early weeks of pregnancy.

> If you are overweight, you should lose the extra pounds before you become pregnant. Dieting while pregnant is not safe because it can deprive the growing child of essential nutrients. If you are underweight, try to gain the additional weight before you conceive so the baby will have the best possible environment.

> Review all of your prescription drugs and over-the-counter medicines with your doctor. Remember to include ALL medications you take regularly, not just the ones prescribed by that doctor. Some drugs are known to cause birth defects, and your doctor may want you to discontinue them at least six weeks before you try to conceive.

> If you have never had German measles (rubella), your doctor may recommend taking a rubella vaccine shot. If you get German measles while you are pregnant, you would be at high risk of having a baby with birth defects. Therefore, the vaccine should be taken *before* you are pregnant.

> If you have been taking oral contraceptives,

doctors recommend using barrier-contraceptives for at least two cycles before you try to become pregnant. Obstetrics specialist, Dr. Roy Pitkin from the University of Iowa, explains that taking oral contraceptives leads to a deficiency of the vitamin folic acid which is important for fetal development. This two-month period, combined with a proper diet, will allow the woman's body to build up adequate folic acid supplies, Pitkin suggests. Folic acid supplements taken before and during pregnancy can cut birth defects.

> Eat a well-balanced diet or take a daily multi-vitamin while you are trying to conceive. A good diet will provide adequate nourishment for the child in the first weeks before you know you are pregnant. Calcium, zinc and iron are especially important. Avoid megadoses of vitamins. Many vitamins and minerals can be dangerous in high doses. The Recommended Daily Dietary Allowance (RDA) suggested for pregnant women is all the vitamins and minerals you will need for a healthy baby.

> Reduce or eliminate your intake of coffee and other products high in caffeine because caffeine has been linked to a higher risk of spontaneous abortions (miscarriages).

> When you are trying to get pregnant, avoid

alcohol after you ovulate until you start your period. The development of the baby in the first few days after conception is very important. Since the fetus is so small, even a small amount of alcohol could be damaging. Fathers should also avoid heavy drinking in the pre-conception stages. A recent study has linked low birth weights to fathers who drank heavily just prior to conception. (In this study, heavy drinking was defined as two drinks daily or more than four drinks at one time).

> Quit smoking before you conceive. Smoking has been linked to birth defects, decreased fertility, poor growth, spontaneous abortions and stillbirths.

Premenstrual Syndrome (PMS)

•• Over 150 symptoms have been connected to premenstrual syndrome, commonly known as PMS, reports the Health and Nutrition Newsletter (1:12) from Columbia University. PMS symptoms occur during the last 10 days before the menstrual period begins and stop within a week after the start of the period. Some of the most common symptoms according to Columbia University are:

> anxiety
> bloating of the stomach
> bowel cramping

> breast swelling and tenderness
> change in sex drive
> constipation
> crying spells
> depression
> diarrhea
> dizziness
> forgetfulness
> frequent urination
> headache
> increased appetite
> low blood sugar
> migraine headache
> mood swings
> rapid heartbeats
> restlessness
> sleep problems
> tiredness
> water retention

•• The more coffee you drink the more severe your PMS symptoms become, according to research in the <u>American</u> <u>Journal</u> <u>of</u> <u>Public</u> <u>Health</u> (75: 11,1335). Women with the most severe PMS problems were found to drink four or more cups of coffee daily. Despite this discovery, many over-the-counter products for PMS symptoms contain caffeine. Read the labels and don't use products containing caffeine to treat your PMS symptoms.

•• Dr. Susan Lark, author of <u>The</u> <u>Premenstrual</u> <u>Syndrome</u> <u>Self-Help</u> <u>Book</u>, suggests eliminating coffee and making other dietary changes to reduce PMS problems.

> Eliminate pork, beef and lamb because they lead to an increase in the body's production of estrogen, Lark says.

> Eliminate alcohol. Like the above meats, alcohol causes the body to produce more estrogen and should be avoided.

> Eliminate sugar to help reduce mood swings caused by changing blood-sugar levels. Avoid chocolate because it increases the craving for sweets.

> Eliminate foods high in sodium which lead to water retention and bloating.

> Eliminate dairy products because they interfere with the body's absorption of calcium, explains Lark. Proper absorption of magnesium is important to reduce PMS.

•• Some over-the-counter products are available to help relieve PMS symptoms. According to a review of available drugs by the Food and Drug Administration (FDA), over-the-counter products, which include these drugs, are safe and effective for their stated purpose:

> Ammonium chloride, pamabrom and pyrilamine maleate for water retention and bloating.

> Aspirin, acetaminophen, and ibuprofen for cramps, lower back pain and headaches.

> Pyrilamine maleate for mood changes.

•• Tranquilizers available only by prescription and taken for two weeks prior to menstruation seem to help relieve some of the tension some women experience.

•• Since PMS is caused by the hormonal changes in a woman's body just prior to menstruation, hormonal drugs have been used to fight PMS problems. However, according to the Mayo Clinic Health Letter (5:2) birth control pills cause PMS problems in about the same number of women as they help.

•• Painful, lumpy breasts can be caused by PMS or could be a sign of cancer. If the breast pain is worst just prior to menstruation and goes away as soon as the period starts, the breasts are usually not cancerous, says Dr. Susan Love, director of Beth Israel Hospital's breast clinic. Any severe breast pain or lumps should be reported to your doctor, Dr. Love suggests. Breast pain in women who have already gone through menopause should be reported immediately.

•• Evening primrose oil was found to help relieve painful breasts experienced just prior to menstruation in 45% of women. Evening primrose oil, often sold in health-food stores is high in unsaturated fatty acids like lineolic acid. According to the British study, the oil must be taken daily for three months to be effective for painful breasts.

•• Cut down the amount of fat in your regular diet. Low-fat diets have been shown to reduce pain in breasts prior to menstruation, two recent studies report.

•• Dr. Michael Osborne at Memorial Sloan-Kettering in New York suggests that women with painful breasts due to PMS should wear a supportive bra to bed each night and take over-the-counter painkillers when needed.

Pressure Sores

•• Pressure sores or bed sores are caused when a person must lie in bed for long periods of time. Patients recuperating from a serious illness or accident are most likely to develop them. Sores develop on the areas where the body has the most pressure. In their initial stages, bed sores are just annoying, but left unnoticed or untreated they can become very serious problems that jeopardize overall health.

•• Application of cod liver oil, castor oil, granulated sugar, ice packs, linseed oil, cornstarch, egg whites or honey has been suggested for home treatment of bed sores. Unfortunately, none of these methods has been medically proven to be effective. In fact, some of these remedies may promote yeast or bacterial infections of the sores. The best treatment for bed sores is to remove the pressure on the area and treat the sore with antibiotic ointment.

•• Prevention is much better than trying to find a suitable treatment. Take steps to prevent bed sores from occurring. A person who must stay in bed for several days should be turned at least every two hours. Use a water mattress, air bed, air mattress, foam rubber mat or a sheepskin pad to help reduce the occurrence of pressure sores. Bed sheets should be kept loose, and the person should be kept dry. Excess sweating or incontinence increases the chances of pressure sores developing. Never raise the head of the bed because this causes additional pressure on the lower part of the body which can lead to pressure sores.

Safe Sex

•• "Safe sex" has become a widespread topic since the development of the AIDS virus and other sexually transmitted diseases. The best way to prevent sexually transmitted diseases is to have only one partner, your spouse. Any other sexual activity should be considered a high risk. The use of condoms is being advocated to help prevent these diseases, but they are not 100% guaranteed "safe". In a recent study, condoms failed in over 25% of the times they were used.

Skin Problems

•• The proper climate may help relieve stubborn cases of psoriasis, reports the Journal of the American Academy of Dermatology. The Dead Sea in Israel seems to have the best combination of climate and location. This site has a low altitude that helps filter out the harmful rays of the sun, and the Dead Sea has a high mineral and salt content. In 85% of the cases where psoriasis sufferers sunbathe and take daily dips in the mineral-laden water, the psoriasis completely disappears or greatly improves within four weeks of treatment. Psoriasis is often inactive for six months after treatment and is usually milder if it returns, according to the Journal.

•• Serious skin problems can contribute to a poor self-image which can lead to depression, warns Dr. Thomas F. Cash at Old Dominion University in Norfolk, Virginia. Many people with skin problems start to feel that people are looking at them or that they are not acceptable to others.

•• Exposure to the sun's ultraviolet rays can increase the incidence of "latent" skin problems like cold sores and warts, confirms Mary Norval at the University of Edinburgh in Scotland. The research team there discovered that exposure to ultraviolet light actually diminishes the protective antibodies in the skin and allows such problems to flourish. Sudden, excessive exposure to the sun is the worst threat. Norval suggests that people who are not used to being in the sun should wear a maximum protection sunblock (SPF 15) when they are exposed.

•• Tanning with sunlamps or in tanning salons that use just ultraviolet "A" rays may be more dangerous than tanning with the sun, reports the Archives of Dermatology (119:641). The damage leading to skin cancer is believed to be caused by the medium ultraviolet "B" rays, therefore tanning lamps using only ultraviolet "A" rays were thought to be safe. However, according to the journal report, when skin is exposed to regular sunshine after being exposed to just the ultraviolet "A" rays, the skin becomes severely damaged. The researchers believe that the combination actually increases the risk of developing skin cancer. They urge people to avoid ultraviolet "A" sunlamps.

•• Exposure to ultraviolet rays is known to contribute to skin cancer, wrinkling, and early aging. With the gradual depletion of the ozone layer, the protective layer of the earth's atmosphere, and with the increasing popularity of sunbathing, doctors warn that the development of skin cancer is on the rise. In 1982, one out of every 250 people developed skin cancer. But by the year 2000, one out of every 90 will develop it, forecasts Dr. Darrel Rigel of the New York University Medical Center.

•• Learn to protect your skin:

> Always use a sunscreen. The Food and Drug Administration explains that sunscreens rated with a SPF (sun protection factor) of 2-4 offer only minimal protection; 4-6 is moderate protection; 8-15 maximal; and over 15 is considered ultra protection. There is only a slight difference between the protective power of a 15 and a 23 SPF-rated lotion, so consumer advocates recommend 15 SPF.

> Apply the sunscreen on all exposed skin.

> The sunscreen is most effective if you apply it 15 minutes to an hour BEFORE exposing yourself to the sun. Putting on the sunscreen prior to exposure allows maximum protection because the chemicals have time to properly penetrate the skin.

> Use a sunscreen that contains PABA (para-aminobenzoic acid) because it helps to absorb the harmful rays.

> Re-apply sunscreen after swimming or getting wet with perspiration. Waterproof sunscreen products should protect you for at least 80 minutes of swimming or sweating. Water-resistant products should protect you for at least 30 minutes. But if you towel off after swimming or sweating, you will remove the screen. Re-apply sunscreen after using a towel.

> Remember that the sun's ultraviolet rays can penetrate through three feet of water. If you are snorkeling, surfing, swimming, or participating in any water sports, be sure to wear a waterproof sunscreen. Even though you may not feel the heat while in the water, your skin could be severely damaged.

> Wear a hat.

> Wear sunglasses.

> It you are really sensitive to the sun, but you enjoy swimming, use a waterproof sunscreen and wear a dark T-shirt over your bathing suit while you are in the water. Re-apply the sunscreen after swimming, even if it is waterproof.

> Do not wear loose-knit bathing suits or "unsuits" that let the ultraviolet rays through the suit's material. "Unsuits" are made from special types of cotton fibers that are not see-through, but they let ultraviolet rays through so people tan even when wearing bathing suits. Loose-knit suits or "unsuits" will allow very sensitive skin, including the pubic areas, to be exposed to ultraviolet rays which could be very damaging.

> The FDA suggests that you check with your pediatrician before applying sunscreen rated higher than 4 on children under two years of age. Do not allow infants to be exposed to direct sunlight.

> Beware of increased exposure to ultraviolet rays when you are in high altitudes or places close to the equator.

> Doctors suggest that everyone, especially people who spend a lot of time outdoors in the sunshine or people who are fair-skinned, should regularly examine themselves for warning signs of skin cancer including: a change in the color or size of a wart or mole; a sore that will not heal or is slow to heal; or a thickening or lump in the breast,

lip, tongue or elsewhere. Active sunbathers, farmers, lifeguards, outdoor construction workers and sailors need to be particularly careful.

> Dangerous exposure to ultraviolet rays is not limited to the summer months. Be careful when participating in winter sports like skiing, ice skating and snowmobiling because the sun's rays are reflected by the snow and exposure to them is intensified.

•• Facial flushing can be eased by sucking on ice cubes, suggests Dr. Johnathon Wilkin at McGuire Veterans Hospital in Richmond, Virginia. Many people suffer facial flushing from drinking hot drinks, getting excited or angered, or from menopause. By sucking on ice cubes, the blood in the neck area is cooled and the flushing stops, Wilkin explains.

•• If you exercise regularly and suffer from skin problems in the areas where you perspire, carry your own cleanser. Apply an astringent skin cleanser to some cotton balls or a small towel. Place them in a plastic bag and carry them with you while you exercise. When you feel the sweat starting to flow, wipe the area clean with your cleanser.

•• To end dry skin:

> Drink eight glasses of water a day. The

water will help your entire body, including keeping your skin moist, preventing dehydration, and helping to flush out waste materials.

> Do not overbathe. Shower or bathe only every second day. Between baths, try a sponge bath to clean under your arms, your rectum and your pubic area, which need to be cleaned daily. Excessive showering dries out the skin unnecessarily.

> Use cool or lukewarm water. Hot water dries out the skin more than cool water.

> Avoid heavily scented soaps. Fragrances can contribute to overly dry skin.

> For best results, prepare your skin before using a moisturizer. Allow your pores to open up by putting a towel dampened with warm water on your skin for five minutes. Then apply your moisturizer. Your skin will be more receptive to the moisturizer after the warm towel treatment.

> For a simple, inexpensive moisturizing treatment, apply a layer of petroleum jelly or shortening, then cover the area with plastic wrap for several hours.

> Dr. Diana Bihova, a skin specialist who teaches at New York University Medical Center, recommends moisturizers that contain urea or lactic acid. Remember that the price of the

moisturizer is not a reflection of how effective it will be. Check the labels.

> To avoid dry legs, Adrian Arpel recommends shaving with sunflower, peanut, almond or sesame oil rather than shaving cream.

•• Oil in the skin and hair may be reduced by lowering the amount of fats in your diet, according to Jackie Rogers of the Life Control Institute in Phillipsburg, New Jersey. To learn more about how to reduce the amount of fat in a daily diet, see our report on **Cholesterol Reduction** in this book.

•• Wrinkles are a sign of graceful aging, but premature wrinkles can be prevented by good skin care:

> Do not smoke. A study published in the British Medical Journal showed that wrinkles around the eyes and lips, odd colored complexions, dry skin and leathery skin are more likely to occur in heavy smokers. Other studies have shown that the physical action of drawing in the smoke through pursed lips creates hollow cheeks. Smoking also decreases the circulation of blood which is necessary for healthy skin. A spokesperson for SmokEnders, a respected quit-smoking program, claims that if you quit smoking, your skin will improve.

> Avoid quick weight loss or gain. Sudden changes in body weight damage the elasticity of the skin and eventually cause wrinkles. Gradual weight loss or gain is better for your skin and entire body.

> Eat a healthful diet. Include foods rich in vitamins A, B, C, D, selenium and zinc for the most wrinkle-free skin.

> Exercise regularly. According to Women's Day (3/3/87), studies have shown that athletes' skin contains more collagen and is thicker than nonathletes. Collagen is an important factor in preventing wrinkles. Exercise is thought to help promote skin cell growth and improve the blood circulation.

> Don't strain or overuse your facial muscles. Wearing protective sunglasses can prevent unnecessary squinting. Corrective glasses may stop you from straining your eyes and facial muscles. Massage your facial muscles gently during intense periods of concentration.

> Practice stress reduction in your life. Stress can often affect how tightly we hold our faces and cause wrinkles. Teach yourself to relax your facial muscles when dealing with stress. Learning to relax can improve the looks of your skin. Also see our report on **Stress** in this book.

> Avoid drastic changes in temperature. In extremely cold weather, expose as little skin as possible by wearing a scarf and dressing properly.

> Avoid exposure to ultraviolet rays from the sun or artificial tanning lights.

> Do not sleep on your side or with your face on your pillow. Sleeping on your back will prevent your face from being pushed into your pillow which causes wrinkles.

> Moisturize your skin regularly. Nothing has been proven to actually stop your skin from aging, but moisturizers will help your skin to feel smooth and soft.

> Skin care experts recommend exfoliating your skin regularly. Exfoliating is the process where dead skin cells are removed, either with a commercial preparation (masks or scrubs) or by rubbing your face with a towel. Experts believe that exfoliating helps the skin to produce new cells which improves the skin's appearance.

> Be careful with your use of cosmetics. According to the FDA, there have not been any studies on the long-term effects of cosmetic use. When cosmetics are used, be sure to cleanse your skin at the end of each day. It may be wise to avoid using any cosmetics at least a few days a month to allow your skin to "breathe".

Sleep Problems

•• Here are some tips for better sleep from the American Narcolepsy Association.

> Accept occasional bouts with sleeplessness. Lack of sleep is often a response to stress or a crisis. Don't fret over these occasional experiences. Some people worry so much about "being afraid that they may not fall asleep" that they actually create insomnia.

> Recognize that eight hours of sleep each night is not essential for every adult. Some people find they require more than eight hours, and some do well with less. Many older adults find that they need less sleep. Get only as much sleep as you need because staying in bed for longer periods than necessary may lead to shallow, unsatisfactory sleep.

> Establish a regular time to go to bed and a regular wake-up time even if you sleep poorly. Regular bedtimes and waking times, including weekends, may help sleeping problems. However, remember that some people seem to be night owls, and some are "morning" people, depending on their unique biological clocks. Experiment with different schedules until you feel that you are

sleeping and rising at the best times for your body.

> If you are not sleepy, leave your bed and your bedroom. Do some peaceful activity, then return to bed when you are tired. Try to keep your bed as a place for sleep and not for tossing, turning or worrying about falling asleep.

> Create a good atmosphere for a restful sleep — quiet, dark, and with a comfortable temperature. If noise from traffic, airplanes, animals or other people disturbs your sleep, make your bedroom as quiet as possible. Use heavy drapes, turn a radio on low, or keep a fan or air-conditioner on for a constant sound level. Some stores sell products that use only a small amount of electricity and are made expressly to drown out unwanted noises. One brand called "Sleepmate" is available at many retail stores. Use ear plugs only as a last resort, especially if you live alone, because you would not be able to hear in case of an emergency. A room that is too light may also cause problems. Curtains, blinds or a blindfold can help keep out light. A room that is too hot or too cold may inhibit sleep. Be sure to have the room temperature comfortable for your needs. Use layers of bedding, so one layer can be easily removed or added as needed during the night.

> Do not use over-the-counter sleep aids. You

may become dependent on them, and their effectiveness is reduced with long-term use. Drugs that promote sleep may prevent sleep from progressing into its normal varying stages which could cause other health and psychological problems. Using "sleeping pills" may be medically dangerous if you are a heavy sleeper, experience sleeplessness during the day, or have sleep apnea. Sleep apnea is a serious condition when a person temporarily stops breathing during sleep.

> Avoid chronic use of alcohol because it leads to disturbed sleep and is addictive.

> Reduce or eliminate use of caffeine, nicotine or other stimulants during the day.

> Don't go to bed hungry. A small snack, like a piece of fruit, may help calm hunger pangs and provide better sleep.

> Avoid a sedentary lifestyle. Regular exercise and activity will help increase your ability to fall asleep easily.

> Listening to music with the same amount of beats per minute as a relaxed heart beat (about 68 beats per minute) may be helpful, suggests Cheryl Sedei-Godley, a music therapist from Florida. Once you find a piece of music that is peaceful and helps you fall asleep, use it regularly as part of your sleep routine.

> Biofeedback has successfully been used to treat sleeplessness. Biofeedback is a technique taught in certain clinics that teaches you to control certain body functions allowing you to relax for sleep.

> Depression can cause an inability to sleep. If someone displays signs of depression, treating the depression may help overcome the sleep problem. Also see **Depression** in this book.

> Other medical problems can cause an inability to sleep, including indigestion, asthma, headaches, arthritis, angina, epilepsy or other pains. If you suspect that your sleeplessness may be caused by a medical problem, be sure to see your doctor.

•• Snoring is associated with sleep apnea, a dangerous problem when someone temporarily stops breathing during sleep. According to the Food and Drug Administration (FDA), overweight men seem to suffer from sleep apnea more than any other group. People with sleep apnea score about ten points lower than normal on IQ tests because the condition affects their ability to concentrate and remember, reports the journal Sleep (June 1987).

Loud snoring or severe snoring episodes associated with gaps in breathing should be reported to your doctor. If you suspect sleep apnea, do not take sleeping pills, tranquilizers, over-the-counter sleeping products or cold medicines as they could alter your body's ability to start breathing again. Sleep apnea can be fatal, so self-treatment is not recommended. Work with your doctor to overcome this problem.

Signs of sleep apnea which should be reported to your physician (FDA Consumer 20:10) include:
> not feeling awake or rested after sleeping
> snoring
> waking up breathless or with a snort in the middle of a sleepful period
> daytime sleepiness
> sleepwalking
> observation by another person that you stop breathing during your sleep
> hallucinations
> irritability
> bedwetting
> a short, thick neck
> blackouts
> senility
> poor concentration
> loss of interest in sex
> personality changes
> irrational behavior
> morning headaches

•• To relieve sleep apnea, your doctor may suggest:
> losing weight
> sleeping on two pillows
> raising the head of the bed by six inches
> sleeping in a reclining chair
> not sleeping on your back . . . by sewing a large marble, tennis ball or other object in the back of the pajamas, at the spine just below the neck.
> surgically removing the tonsils or adenoids
> using a Continuous Positive Airway Pressure (CPAP) device that must be prescribed by a doctor. This machine is attached to the nose of a person with sleep apnea and gently applies constant air pressure during the night so breathing will not be interrupted. According to the FDA, the device is effective in about 85% of sleep apnea patients.

•• According to Dr. Andrew Aronfy of Greenbelt, Maryland, there are several causes of sleep problems in children which vary according to the age of the child. During infancy (birth to eight months) sleeplessness is caused by physical problems. A small baby has a small stomach and needs to eat every three to four hours around the clock. In addition, the baby may have colic, or a diaper rash, or may be uncomfortable in some other way. Treatment should be directed towards finding the cause and correcting it.

Between eight months and three years, sleep problems are more complicated; so are the solutions, says Dr. Aronfy. Physical causes may still be present, but now emotional problems predominate.

> SEPARATION ANXIETY is a major issue. The child wishes to remain near the parents at all times. Separation produces fear, and fear results in sleeplessness. A night-light in the bedroom and the door slightly ajar may solve this problem. When the child hears his parents moving around and talking in another room, he will be reassured and fall asleep.

> The most frequent cause in this age group is simply HABIT. Here the child has no trouble falling asleep, but he will wake up one or more times in the middle of the night. He will then roam around the house, or climb in bed with his parents. To treat this condition, make sure there are no obvious problems (fever, pain, hunger, nightmares, uncomfortable surroundings, etc.) If no such problems exist, talk to the child soothingly, but do NOT pick him up, coddle him, or feed him. If you have to, stay in his room until he falls asleep. If later he gets out of bed and sleeps on the floor or

on a chair, that is all right. If he climbs in bed with you, take him back to his bed as often as necessary. You must be more stubborn than he is! For the first few nights you may not get much sleep, but after that the habit will be broken, if you persevere.

Sleep disturbances in children over three years have causes more like adults: worry, illness, fear, family problems, overstimulation, change of environment, etc. The sleep problem disappears when the cause is resolved. The child must be told that he need not go to sleep, and need not stay in bed, but he must stay in his room and not disturb others, says Dr. Aronfy.

Sneezing

•• Sneezing is an important body function that should not be stifled or stopped. The American Journal of Otolaryngology reports that pinching the nostrils closed during a sneeze causes damage to the inner ear. The closed nostrils may also force the mucus into the ear canals and cause ear infections.

However, the nose should be covered with a handkerchief or facial tissue to help prevent the spread of germs. If the hands are used to cover the nose, they should be thoroughly washed immediately after the sneeze. It is preferable to cover the nose with the hands rather than leaving the nose uncovered during a sneeze.

Stress

•• Stress specialists and the National Mental Health Association suggest these methods to help deal with your tensions:

> Do something physical to deal with tension or anger. Many people find that studying the martial arts, kneading bread, gardening or exercising helps release tension, making them more able to deal with the situation.

> Simple deep breathing exercises or gentle neck rolls may help relax the neck and body.

> Remember to take one day at a time. Worrying about the future may be overwhelming, but dealing with only today's problems may be within our capabilities.

> During times of crisis or great change, keep some things routine. Normal routines will provide a refuge in the midst of great stress. Do not make important decisions during stressful times because stress can distort your understanding of what may be best.

> Take time for yourself. You've heard this

before but actually achieving it may be difficult. If you are busy, try scheduling time for yourself each day. Your time could be physical exercise or mental exercise like reading or enjoying theatre. If you schedule it and make it important, you should find the other problems easier to cope with.

> Take vacations that are good for you. A long vacation is often prescribed to relieve stress, but some people return to work to find more stress, due to piled-up work, than when they left. If you do not have someone to do your job while you are away, you may want to consider taking short vacations, like extended weekends, rather than missing one or more weeks at a time.

> Concentrate on praise rather than criticism. If you are always looking for the worst, you will usually find it. You will be tense because situations don't meet your standards. Practice finding something good in every situation.

> Forgive. If you forgive a rude waitress or fellow commuter, you will release tension. Forgiving them and letting the incident go will be calming.

> Don't be competitive with other people at times when it is not appropriate. In our highly competitive society, it is sometimes difficult to stop that competitiveness from creeping into our

private lives. For example, when driving, it is NOT important to see how many people you can pass. This type of activity adds unnecessary tension to your life.

> Take notes and write down important things. Your notes can act as a "security blanket" that allows you to feel calm because you have a record of all the times and necessary details.

> Consider getting a dog as a pet. A study at Indiana University found that couples that had dogs experienced fewer marital problems and less stress. The dogs were found to be "soothing" and allowed the couples to deal better with the stresses in their marriage and their lives.

> Using mental images is a healthy way to "escape" from tension and relax for a few minutes. Doctors suggest closing your eyes and picturing a very peaceful scene in your "mind's eye". Go back to your favorite resting spot, perhaps a place by a clear-flowing stream. Picture every detail, hear the birds and smell the flowers. Imagining will help you relax so you can cope with the tension at hand.

> Lying on a sheepskin on a water mattress inside a "float tank" may help relieve stress, according to Dr. Lloyd Glauberman of New York (Health 19:2). Dr. Glauberman plays audio tapes

for the person in the float tank which include subliminal messages on stress reduction. He finds that the tank helps the psychologist when dealing with stress.

> According to Georgia Witkin-Lanoil, Ph.D., author of The Male Stress Syndrome, you need to recognize your own response to stress so you can then release the tension. Dr. Witkin-Lanoil found that women living with men recognized the man's stress responses long before the man was aware of the stress. Women found that men under stress are defensive, disorganized, irritable, aggressive while driving, oversensitive, defiant, and tend to withdraw from their familes. Physically the men experienced stiff necks, indigestion, lack of sleep, nausea, backaches, headaches and allergies while under stress. The women in the home noticed their man's physical symptoms while the men were not as aware of their own stress signals. Dr. Witkin-Lanoil suggests that couples support each other during times of stress and that men should listen to their partners' warnings about being overstressed.

Stroke
•• Eating fresh fruit and vegetables daily could decrease your risk of having a stroke by up to 40%,

according to a new study published in The New England Journal of Medicine 316:235-40). Potassium, found in many fruits and vegetables, may be the difference, say the researchers. Potassium helps lower blood pressure levels; high blood pressure is the leading factor in strokes. Potatoes, raisins, tomatoes, bananas, avocados, orange juice, apricots, squash and cantaloupe are all good sources of potassium.

•• Stop smoking. Smoking has been proven to increase the risk of stroke, reports The New England Journal of Medicine (315:717-20). After a person gives up smoking for at least five years, the risk of having a stroke will drop to about the same level as that of a nonsmoker.

•• Avoid alcohol. A study by researchers in Birmingham, England, showed that men with heavy alcohol consumption have an increased risk of stroke (The New England Journal of Medicine 315:1041-6).

Sunburn

•• To relieve sunburn:

> Take aspirin.

> Soak in cool water or apply cold compresses directly to the sunburned skin. Do not apply any

lotion that will block the pores because the heat will be retained rather than released.

> HCA Grand Strand General Hospital in Myrtle Beach, South Carolina, recommends cool compresses soaked in fluid containing one cup of vinegar to one gallon of ice water, or two ounces of cool Milk of Magnesia mixed with four aspirin.

> If using an aloe gel or other cream to help alleviate sunburn, store it in the refrigerator or on ice.

> Be careful when using lotions containing benzocaine because many people are allergic to it. The allergic reaction could be worse than the sunburn.

> Go to a doctor or emergency clinic if the skin becomes blistered or raw.

•• Avoiding sunburn completely is the best solution to this problem. For tips on how to use sunscreens and prevent sunburn, see our report on **Skin Problems** in this book.

Sunstroke

•• Sunstroke can be caused by over-exposure to the sun and its drying heat. Symptoms include fever, nausea, dizziness, dry skin and fast pulse. To relieve sunstroke:

> Get the victim out of the sun as soon as possible. Have him lie down with head raised.

> Give the person cool (not too cold) liquids to drink. Do not overload with liquids.

> Apply cool compresses on the forehead and at the back of the neck.

> If sunburn has also occurred, have the person soak in a cool tub of water.

•• To avoid sunstroke, take the same precautions as you take against sunburn, plus drinking lots of fluids, especially water. When outdoors, try to avoid direct sunlight and wear a hat and protective, loose clothing.

Swimmer's Ear

•• Swimmer's ear is a common ear infection caused by small organisms in the ear canal. Once swimmer's ear occurs, the doctor should be consulted for antibiotics.

•• To prevent swimmer's ear:

> Avoid swimming in ponds or slow-moving bodies of water.

> Completely dry your ears after swimming, diving or washing, but do NOT use cotton-tipped swabs as they can cause ear damage and infections. You can gently dry the outer part of the ear with a

towel. Shake your head or tilt it to one side to drain any water out of the ears. Fan your ears dry with your hands or a hair dryer on a low setting.

> After swimming, place a solution of equal parts of rubbing alcohol and vinegar in the ear canal to help restore the natural acid level, according to <u>Physician</u> <u>and</u> <u>Sportsmedicine</u> (14:11,57). If you are allergic to alcohol, you can use water and vinegar instead. This solution can be used three times a day to help fight the infection until you can see a doctor. Antibiotics prescribed by a doctor will be the most effective treatment.

Taste — Loss of

•• Long-term use of smokeless tobacco, like chewing tobacco and snuff, "may reduce taste sensitivity and . . . alter preferences for sweet, salty and bitter solutions," according to Dr. David J. Mela of the Monell Chemical Senses Center (<u>The</u> <u>New</u> <u>England</u> <u>Journal</u> <u>of</u> <u>Medicine</u> 316: 18, 1165-66).

•• Zinc supplements may improve the sense of taste, according to <u>Vitamin</u> <u>Side</u> <u>Effects</u> <u>Revealed</u>. Anorexia nervosa, a serious loss of appetite, has been successfully treated with zinc supplements. High doses of zinc can be dangerous, but eating foods rich in zinc or taking 15 milligrams of zinc a day could improve the sense of taste. Liver, seafood, dairy products, meat and eggs are good natural sources of zinc.

Teeth See: **Dental Problems**

Toxic Shock Syndrome (TSS)

•• Toxic Shock Syndrome can occur in men and children but most often occurs in women. High fever, diarrhea, skin rash, vomiting, blurred vision, disorientation or shock are the symptoms. If TSS is suspected, the person should be rushed to the hospital immediately. TSS is often experienced during menstruation or immediately after.

•• Even though bacteria can enter the body by other ways, most cases of TSS have been linked to use of vaginal tampons during menstruation, reports the medical journal <u>Surgery</u> (March 1987). To reduce your chances of getting toxic shock, doctors recommend:

> Replace tampons every three to four hours and follow all instructions included in the package.

> If possible, alternate using tampons and pads.

> Do not sleep with a tampon in place.

> Do not use superabsorbent tampons. The Food and Drug Administration (FDA) recommends using the "least absorbent tampon" to meet your needs.

> Women who have just given birth or had vaginal surgery, like a D&C (dilatation and curettage), should avoid using tampons for at least two weeks following surgery.

> Women using the contraceptive sponge, Today®, should be alerted to the possibility of developing TSS, especially when the contraceptive sponge is not completely removed from the vagina. All directions on the package should be followed carefully for safest use.

Ulcers
•• Plantains, a type of banana commonly found in developing countries, may help heal gastric ulcers, report some British researchers. Raw plantains seem to stimulate the growth of new stomach cells which helps the ulcers heal, reports Ralph Best at the University of Aston in England. It seems that heat destroys the healing chemical, so Best recommends eating the plantain raw or cooked slowly at a low temperature.

•• Smokers may find that their ulcers begin to heal when they quit smoking.

Vocal Problems   See: Hoarseness

Weight Loss Tips

•• Being more than 15% overweight can lead to many health problems including joint disease, coronary artery disease, stroke, high blood pressure, high cholesterol levels, diabetes, gallstones, gouty arthritis, osteoarthritis, cancer, skin problems, breathing difficulties, sleep apnea, kidney disease, increased risk during surgery, increased risk of complications during pregnancy, and a delay in the discovery of abdominal diseases.

•• If you are over 60 years old, need to lose 20 pounds or more, or have an immediate family member who has had a heart attack or diabetes, consult your doctor before starting on ANY weight loss program.

•• Here are some tips on how to change your eating habits so you can lose weight and keep it off:

> Avoid crash diets and dangerous weight-loss schemes. Choose a diet that you can live with for

the rest of your life. Once someone goes off a severe diet, they usually binge to meet all their cravings that have not been fulfilled. Cycles of rapid weight loss, weight gain, weight loss and weight gain are extremely hard on the body's organs, can lead to high blood pressure and can be dangerous to your overall health. Gradual weight loss that can be maintained is the healthiest way to lose weight.

> Keep a food journal of what, how much and when you eat each day. With a journal you can see exactly where your calories and nutrition are coming from and how you can alter your eating habits.

> Weigh yourself once a week and record it in your food journal. Daily fluctuations in weight are not reliable, but a weekly weighing will allow you to evaluate if your program is working.

> Set a realistic goal weight for yourself, preferably with your doctor's endorsement. Being overweight is dangerous, but so is being underweight. Each person has a different metabolism setting that burns calories at slightly different rates. Choose a weight that is safe and healthy for your height, age and lifestyle.

> Choose specific times to eat your meals and snacks, and do not eat at any other time. Never

skip meals because you will be inclined to eat more at the next meal to make up the difference.

> Do not eat if you are not hungry. As children, we were often required to eat "everything on our plates" and to eat even when we were not hungry, but these patterns can lead to obesity.

> Learn to say "no" without feeling guilty. Once again, do not let someone coerce you into eating.

> Eat slowly. Put your utensils down after each bite. It takes several minutes for the stomach to tell the brain that it is full, so eating slowly will help you to realize you're full before you overeat.

> Try to reduce your intake of all food rather than completely restricting yourself to certain foods. If you are not allowed to have a specific item, usually you will crave that "forbidden fruit." This is particularly true when working with overweight children. It is best to learn good overall eating habits rather than prohibiting certain foods for the rest of their lives.

> Drink grapefruit juice, tomato juice or unsweetened lemonade as an appetizer before your meal. If you allow 20 minutes before you eat, the acid in the juice will help you feel full, and you will be able to eat less. Drink the juice of a whole lemon squeezed into a glass of water, twice a day,

for another natural appetite suppressant.

> Serve your meals on smaller plates so they will look fuller.

> Place the food on the plates away from the table. If you bring serving dishes to the table, you will be more tempted to have additional helpings.

> Avoid dishes and table settings that are bright because bright colors may stimulate the appetite.

> Never eat food out of the original container. Take out an appropriate serving and return the container to its proper place. By eating directly out of the container, you are more likely to eat too much.

> Try to leave something on your plate. In some oriental countries this is considered a high compliment because it shows that you have had plenty to eat. If you have been raised to clear your plate and not to "waste food", learning to leave a small portion on your plate will be good for you.

> Switch to lower calorie foods like skim milk and calorie-reduced products.

> Many doctors now recommend avoiding products with artificial sweeteners. Although they seem to be a boon for dieters, some doctors believe that artificial sweeteners increase or maintain the desire for sweets which is not helpful to someone

who is dieting.

New studies show that people who use artificial sweeteners are heavier than those who don't.

> Eat more vegetables and smaller portions of meat, especially red meat.

> Trim all noticeable fat from meat, and remove the skin before eating.

> Eat plenty of high-fiber foods like whole-grain products, beans and vegetables.

> Don't use butter or margarine for cooking. Use a low saturated fat oil like sunflower, safflower, corn, sesame seed, cottonseed, or soybean.

> Use a low calorie, soft-spread alternate to butter. If you use a soft-spread, you'll use less because it spreads easier than butter or margarine.

> Eliminate alcohol because it is high in "empty" calories. Alcohol products contain a lot of calories, but they have no nutritional value.

> Keep healthful snacks available. Try cutting up celery, carrots, broccoli, cauliflower, radishes and whatever other vegetables you like and leaving them in the refrigerator. Buy plenty of fruit. They will be quick and easy snacks.

> Buy high-quality popcorn that tastes good without butter or salt. To flavor your popcorn, try lightly spraying the popcorn with a low calorie

vegetable oil, then add cinnamon, curry powder, onion powder, chili powder or other herbs. (Salt increases water retention, which adds to your weight, so you may want to reduce your salt intake as well as your calories).

> Reduce or eliminate high calorie nuts and nut products, including peanut butter.

> Never go grocery shopping when you are hungry. If you are hungry, you will tend to buy more, and you are more easily tempted to buy high-calorie foods.

> Make a shopping list of things you need and stick to it. Don't be seduced by unnecessary foods.

> Don't keep high-calorie food in your home.

> Don't store food within sight.

> The Good Wellness Program for Weight Management suggests placing a bottle of mouthwash in front of the refrigerator door. If you stray into the kitchen looking for "something to eat", you will have to move the mouthwash first. Rogers, director of the program, suggests rinsing with the mouthwash to satisfy the cravings without consuming any calories.

> Brushing your teeth frequently may help reduce snacking. Your teeth and mouth feel so good that you don't have the desire to eat.

> Remember your diet when eating outside of

your home, at a restaurant, or someone else's home. If you eat at a cafeteria, like a school lunchroom, check with the food services manager to see if low-calorie meals can be special ordered.

> If you must have dessert, try sharing it with one or two other people. After a fine meal, you do not need the dessert, but a small sample may meet your craving for a sweet.

> When flying or traveling by train, request a low-calorie meal at least 24 hours in advance of your departure.

> Do not reward yourself with food or use food to fight stress or depression. Buy yourself a gift or treat yourself to a favorite activity, rather than using food as a release or reward.

> Eating "spicy" foods may help speed up your metabolism and burn up more calories, researchers at Oxford Polytechnic report. In three hours of initial testing, a group of people who ate food spiced with mustard sauce and chili burned up to 76 calories more than people who ate the same food without the spices. The researchers are not sure if the same "high metabolism" will continue if hot foods become part of an everyday diet.

> Do not use over-the-counter appetite suppressants or other diet pills. One common ingredient, phenylpropanolamine hydrochloride (PPA) has been found to cause high blood pressure

even at the recommended doses for weight loss. Anyone with diabetes, heart disease, thyroid disease or high blood pressure should avoid these products containing PPA, recommends the Health Letter (2:1).

> Do not use or purchase a product that promises to reduce or remove fat in one specific body area. Except for specific exercise or cosmetic surgery, one part of your body cannot be reduced.

> Do not use a "body wrap" in hopes of losing weight. The only weight loss that body wraps provide is the loss of sweat which is just temporary. Using body wraps can be harmful because the body's temperature is allowed to escalate.

> Try squeezing your earlobe for sixty seconds before eating. This is an ancient technique of acupressure that may help curb your appetite.

> Exercise. Cutting calories and increasing the amount of daily exercise are the keys to losing weight effectively. Remember that routine activities can make a difference: taking the stairs instead of an elevator, manually switching the TV channels, and washing the dishes by hand all increase your "burning" of calories.

> Participate in and develop hobbies that use

energy and calories like walking, swimming, bowling, skiing, tennis, miniature golf, skating or dancing.

> Obese dieters who lose weight very quickly are at increased risk of developing gallstones, doctors at the Cedars-Sinai Medical Center in Los Angeles report. However, if four aspirin are taken each day, the dieter should not develop gallstones, according to the research. You should discuss the aspirin treatment with your doctor if you are considering a low-calorie diet.

Wrinkles   See: **Skin Problems**